Root Canal Errors: Spot, Fix, and Prevent

From Mistakes to Mastery

By: Dr Pavan Tryambake

Specialist in Conservative Dentistry and Endodontics

PhD scholar (MUHS), Nashik

Founder & Chief Endodontist

Rajdant Dental Care, Nashik, Maharashtra

Made with ♥ on the Notion Press Platform

www.notionpress.com

*To my loving wife, **Dr Mrunal**, and my beloved parents, **Chhaya** and **Dr Rajendra**,*

Thank you for your endless love, support, encouragement, and belief in me. This book would not have been possible without you.

With love and gratitude,

Dr Pavan Rajendra Tryambake

CONTENTS

FOREWORD

Endodontic treatment is a combination of sound biological principles, scientific knowledge, and precise clinical execution. While success depends on following established protocols, the ability to recognise, manage, and prevent procedural errors is equally important for achieving predictable outcomes.

Root Canal Errors: Spot, Fix, and Prevent by **Dr Pavan Rajendra Tryambake** addresses one of the most challenging aspects of clinical endodontics. This book provides a practical and systematic approach to understanding the common errors encountered during root canal treatment, their causes, methods of prevention, and appropriate management strategies. The content is presented clearly and concisely, making it valuable for undergraduate and postgraduate students as well as practising clinicians.

I appreciate Dr Pavan's sincere effort in compiling this work to enhance clinical knowledge and improve patient care. I am confident that this book will serve as a useful reference for dental professionals seeking to strengthen their understanding of endodontic procedures and minimise procedural complications.

I congratulate Dr Pavan Rajendra Tryambake on this commendable achievement and wish him continued success in his academic and professional endeavours.

Dr. Siddhesh Bandekar
MDS Guide, *(Conservative Dentistry & Endodontics)*

Department of Conservative Dentistry & Endodontics
Yogita dental college and hospital, Khed
Ratnagiri, Maharashtra

Date: 3 June 2026

PREFACE

Root canal treatment is one of the most predictable procedures in dentistry when performed with sound biological principles, proper diagnosis, and meticulous clinical technique. However, even the most experienced clinicians may encounter procedural errors and unexpected challenges during treatment. The ability to recognise, prevent, and manage these errors is an essential component of successful endodontic practice.

The idea for this book arose from my clinical experience, academic training, and interactions with undergraduate students, postgraduate residents, and practising dentists. I realised that while numerous textbooks describe the ideal steps of root canal treatment, there are comparatively few resources that focus specifically on the procedural errors encountered in daily practice and their practical management.

This book has been written with the objective of providing a concise, practical, and evidence-based guide to the common errors associated with endodontic treatment. Each chapter discusses the causes, prevention, diagnosis, and management of these complications, enabling readers to approach clinical challenges with greater confidence and competence.

This book is intended for undergraduate and postgraduate dental students, general dental practitioners, and endodontists who wish to strengthen their understanding of procedural mishaps and improve the quality and predictability of their clinical outcomes. I hope that the information presented here will help readers avoid common mistakes, make informed clinical decisions, and ultimately provide better care for their patients.

No book is without limitations, and endodontics continues to evolve as advances in materials, technology, and scientific evidence emerge. I encourage readers to combine the knowledge gained from this book with continuous learning, critical thinking, and sound clinical judgment.

I sincerely hope this book serves as a practical companion on your journey toward excellence in endodontic practice.

Dr Pavan Rajendra Tryambake
MDS – Conservative Dentistry & Endodontics

Date: 5 July 202

ACKNOWLEDGMENTS

With the divine blessings of **Vighnaharta Shri Ganesha**, the remover of all obstacles and the embodiment of wisdom, I humbly present *Root Canal Errors: Spot, Fix, and Prevent*. May His blessings guide every clinician in overcoming the complexities of endodontic treatment and inspire the pursuit of excellence in preserving natural dentition through knowledge, precision, and compassion.

No book is ever written in isolation. *Root Canal Errors: Spot, Fix, and Prevent* is the culmination of years of clinical practice, academic learning, research, and the unwavering support of countless individuals who have shaped my professional journey. It is with immense gratitude that I acknowledge those who made this work possible.

First and foremost, I express my deepest gratitude to my beloved parents, **Dr Rajendra Tryambake** and **Mrs Chhaya Tryambake**, whose unconditional love, sacrifices, values, and constant encouragement have been the foundation of my life and career. Their blessings, guidance, and unwavering belief in me have inspired every milestone I have achieved.

My heartfelt appreciation goes to my beloved wife, **Dr Mrunal Tryambake**, whose endless patience, understanding, love, and encouragement sustained me throughout this journey. Her unwavering support during long clinical hours, late-night writing sessions, and demanding academic commitments made the completion of this book possible.

I am equally grateful to my sister, **Dr Komal Tryambake**, and my brother-in-law, **Dr Abhijit Shinde**, for their love, encouragement, and constant faith in my abilities. Their support has always been a source of strength and motivation.

I owe a profound debt of gratitude to my respected teachers and mentors. My sincere thanks to **Prof. Dr Siddhesh Bandekar**, my MDS Guide, whose exceptional mentorship, clinical expertise, and commitment to excellence laid the foundation of my understanding of Endodontics. I am deeply grateful to **Prof. Dr Meenal Gulve**, my PhD Guide, for her invaluable guidance, research mentorship, and continuous encouragement throughout my academic journey. I also extend my sincere appreciation to **Prof. Dr Prashant Moogi**, Head of the Department, for his inspiring leadership, motivation, and constant support.

My heartfelt thanks also go to my respected senior clinicians and mentors—**Dr. Rahul Patil, Dr Santosh Avhad, Dr Shivdas Mhavarkar, and Dr Swapnil Kohle**—whose guidance, clinical insights, and encouragement have significantly contributed to my professional growth and strengthened my passion for Endodontics.

I would also like to express my sincere appreciation to my dear friends and colleagues, whose friendship, encouragement, and shared experiences have enriched both my personal and professional life. My heartfelt thanks to **Dr Kishor Vhorkate, Dr Rahul Sonawane, Dr Akshay Joshi, Dr Prachi Mule, Dr Ravisha Salve, Dr Rohan Garud, Dr Vijay Patil, Dr Deepali Samel, Dr Ved Talathi, Dr Kalyani, Dr Asmita, and Dr Abhijeet Rokade**. Your support, thoughtful discussions, constructive suggestions, and constant encouragement have been invaluable throughout this journey.

I extend my sincere gratitude to my colleagues in the **Indian Dental Association (IDA)** for providing an environment of continuous learning, academic interaction, and professional collaboration. The exchange of ideas and clinical experiences with colleagues has greatly enriched my perspective and reinforced the philosophy behind this book—**Spot, Fix, and Prevent**.

My sincere appreciation goes to the dedicated team at **Rajdant Dental Care, Nashik**. Your professionalism, commitment to patient care, meticulous attention to infection control, and unwavering support allowed me to devote the time and effort necessary to transform years of clinical experience into this book. Working alongside such a dedicated team has been both a privilege and an inspiration.

I am deeply grateful to my patients, who placed their trust and confidence in my hands. Every challenging diagnosis, every complex root canal, every procedural complication, and every successful outcome became an invaluable learning experience. Your faith in me has been the greatest teacher and the true inspiration behind this work.

Finally, I dedicate this book to every undergraduate student, postgraduate resident, general dental practitioner, and endodontist committed to delivering the highest standard of patient care. If the knowledge shared within these pages helps prevent a procedural error, overcome a clinical challenge, restore confidence in a difficult case, or save even a single natural tooth, then this book will have fulfilled its purpose.

I sincerely thank everyone who has directly or indirectly contributed to this journey. Your encouragement, support, and belief in me have made this achievement possible.

May we continue to learn with humility, practice with precision, teach with passion, and preserve natural smiles—one tooth at a time.

Satyameva Jayate.

PROLOGUE/INTRODUCTION

Endodontic errors or procedural accidents are those unfortunate occurrences that happen during treatment, some owing to inattention to detail, others are totally unpredictable.

With the evolution of endodontics, improved instruments and equipment and innovative techniques have contributed to a better quality of treatment. The technological advances have changed the way in which endodontics is practised.[1]

These advancements, in conjunction with increased dental patient education and awareness, have helped to promote the view that the dentition should remain throughout people's lives. As the life span of the population increases, the need to maintain a patient's dentition for a longer period of time has led to a barrage of advanced procedures that were nonexistent years ago. As a result, the need for performing conventional root canal therapy has increased dramatically. This has also led to an increase in the complexity of the cases treated by both general dentists and endodontists. As a result of this, new problems / procedural errors are being created.

Recognition of an error is the first step in its management. After recognition, correction may be accomplished depending on the type and extent of the procedural accident. The next step is to re-evaluate the prognosis of the involved tooth. This is essential as it may affect the entire treatment plan and may also involve dentolegal consequences.[2]

The purpose of this compilation is to present the common endodontic errors and approaches to recognise, correct and prevent them.

Root Canal Errors: Spot, Fix, and Prevent

From Mistakes to Mastery

CLASSIFICATION

Ingle[1] has classified the various endodontic errors based on the procedure during which page they might occur. The classification is as follows:[1]

1. **ACCESS RELATED**
    a. Treating the wrong tooth
    b. Missed canals
    c. Damage to existing restorations
    d. Access cavity perforation
    e. Crown fracture
2. **INSTRUMENTATION RELATED**
    a. Ledge formation
    b. Cervical canal perforation
    c. Mid root perforation
    d. Apical perforation
    e. Separated instruments and foreign objects
    f. Canal blockage
3. **OBTURATION RELATED**
    a. Over or underextended root canal fillings
    b. Neurological complications of endodontic treatment
    c. Vertical root fractures
4. **OTHER ERRORS**
    a. Post space perforation
    b. Irrigant-related errors
    c. Tissue emphysema
    d. Instrument aspiration and ingestion

ACCESS RELATED ERRORS

TREATING THE WRONG TOOTH

Treating the wrong tooth can be due to misdiagnosis or inattention on the part of the dentist.

Misdiagnosis may sometimes happen, and it should not be automatically considered as an endodontic error. This could happen when the patient is not sure of the source of pain, or gives bizarre symptoms, and the radiographic diagnosis is also not conclusive.2

But if one tooth has been diagnosed with a necrotic pulp and if the rubber dam is placed on an adjacent tooth and that tooth is opened, then that is surely a error.3

The problem is recognised, only on reevaluation of the patient, who continues to have symptoms after treatment. Sometimes, the error is detected after the removal of the rubber dam.

First of all, such an error should not be hidden from the patient. Even though it is embarrassing, it is safe to explain the problem to the patient and how it may be corrected.

Appropriate treatment for both teeth should be done, the one incorrectly opened and the one with the original pulpal problem.

Prevention

The endodontist must give attention to detail and obtain as much information from the patient as possible before making the diagnosis. Ingle[1] suggests that, before making a definitive diagnosis, at least three good pieces of evidence should be obtained. These pieces of evidence make a diagnosis of pulp necrosis reasonable and a treatment plan that includes root canal therapy logical.

Tooth marked before isolation.

If less than three pieces of information are available, a definitive diagnosis may not be possible. In such a case, if the patient, who is unable to endure the symptoms, requests to do something, the endodontist may extirpate the pulp as a diagnostic procedure. But the patient should be informed that such a diagnostic procedure also requires completion of root canal therapy, even if it turns out that the problem is with another tooth.

Once a correct diagnosis has been made, the unfortunate situation of opening the wrong tooth can be prevented by marking the tooth to be treated with a pen before isolating it with a rubber dam. [3]

MISSED CANALS

Some root canals are not easily accessible or readily apparent from the chamber. Additional canals in the mesial roots of maxillary molars and distal roots of mandibular molars are good examples of such canals, and these are often left untreated. Other canals are also missed because of a lack of knowledge about root canal anatomy or failure to adequately search for these additional canals. E.g., like lingual canal in mandibular anterior teeth, extra canal in radix entomolaris, etc.[1]

Recognition of a missed canal can occur during or after treatment. During treatment, an instrument or filling material may be noticed to be other than exactly centred in the root, indicating that another canal is present.

In addition to standard radiographs for the determination of missed canals, extra radiographs from mesial and/or distal angulations can be taken. Computerised digital radiography has increased the chances of locating extra canals by enhancing the density and contrast and magnifying the image.

The advent of high-resolution magnification has also increased the ability to locate canals. Magnifying loupes, the microscope, and the endoscope may be used to clinically determine the presence of additional canals.

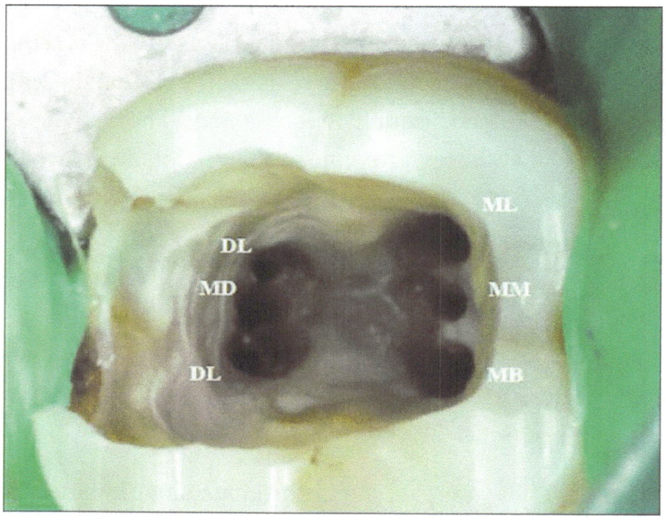

Access to the orifice of all canals

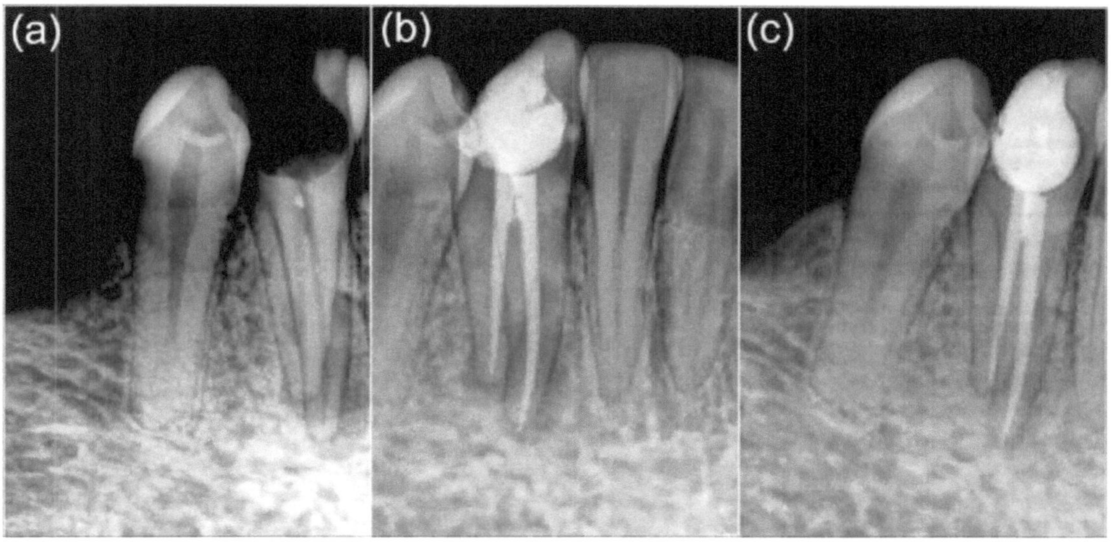

Both canals are obturated in the lower canine.

In some cases, however, recognition may not occur until failure is detected later. In such cases, re-treatment is appropriate and should be attempted before recommending surgical correction.

A missed canal decreases the prognosis and will most likely result in treatment failure. In some teeth with multicanal roots, two canals may have a common apical exit. As long as the apical seal adequately seals both canals, it is possible that the bacterial content in a missed canal may not affect the outcome for some time.

Locating all of the canals in a multi- canal tooth is the best prevention of treatment failure. Adequate coronal access allows the opportunity to find all canal orifices. Any remaining caries and old restorative materials should be removed to provide uncompromised visualisation. Additionally, radiographs taken from mesial and/or distal angles will help to determine if the one canal that has been located is centred in the root, recalling that an eccentrically located canal is highly suggestive of the presence of another canal yet to be found. Knowledge of root canal morphology and knowing which teeth have multiple canals is a good foundation. Assuming at the outset that certain teeth have roots with multiple canals and diligently searching for those canals is a prudent preventive procedure.[4]

DAMAGE TO EXISTING RESTORATION

Access opening is sometimes performed through existing crowns. An existing porcelain or metal crown presents the dentist with additional challenges, like [2]

- Most crowns obscure pulp chamber space on periapical radiographs.
- Root structure or natural crown structure under full coverage restorations may be rotated or malaligned in the normal arch position.
- Most crowns have excessive alloy or composite buildup, which impedes direct access to the opening.
- Visibility into dark access openings in crowns is limited and increases the chance of a error.
- Newer, non-precious alloys are very hard and impede access preparation.
- Access opening through crowns may leave large metallic deposits in the pulp chamber or orifices.
- In preparing an access cavity through a porcelain or porcelain-bonded crown, the porcelain will sometimes chip, or fracture or craze lines may occur even when the most careful approach using water-cooled diamond stones is followed.
- The artificial occlusal or lingual anatomy of a crown restoration does not serve as a guide to access opening.
- Presence of crowns may obscure fractures in the tooth structure, especially the proximal walls or floor of the chamber.
- There is usually no way to predict such an occurrence. Knowing when to exercise caution can, however, reduce unwanted results.[3]

Placing a rubber dam clamp directly on the margin of a porcelain crown is asking for trouble. This may result in damage to the crown margin and/or fracture of the porcelain. In such cases, a clamp can be placed on the adjacent teeth.

If the decision is made to remove the crown for reuse, the visibility is increased, and there is a decrease in the potential for operative error. Despite the various techniques and armamentarium available, the procedure remains unpredictable. If the crown is to be preserved, then a more conservative approach is to be used. Conservative removal efforts are difficult with traditional restorations cemented with nonbonded cements. This situation is more of a concern lately because of the increasing popularity of tooth-colored restorations bonded with adhesive resin restorations.

An alternative to prevent damage to an existing, permanently cemented crown is to remove it before treatment. Even the removal of a provisionally cemented new crown before endodontic therapy may also pose a problem. These crowns can be difficult to remove, and often a margin will be damaged, or the porcelain may chip. Minor porcelain chips can, at times, be repaired by bonding composite resin to the crown. However, the longevity of such repairs is unpredictable.[5]

Various methods of crown removal are:

Preservation of the integrity of the restoration is sometimes possible by using special devices such as the Metalift crown and Bridge Removal system. The system allows for removal with little or no damage to the crown. After completion of root canal therapy, the crown can be recemented and the pilot hole repaired.

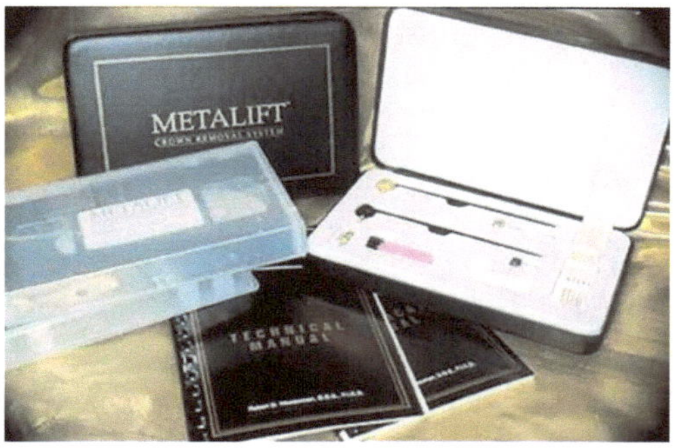

Metalift crown & bridge removal kit

Special forceps, which have been designed specifically for crown removal, can be used. A pair of dental forceps, whether configured for anterior, premolar or molar teeth, includes a pair of jaw-mounted removable cushioning and gripping inserts for conformingly gripping and frictionally retaining a respective dental prosthetic device, such as a crown, to be removed without imposing stress concentrations sufficient to mar or damage the dental prosthetic device.

The Roydent Bridge Remover – designed to specifically engage the margins of the crown while using an adjacent tooth as a fulcrum. Squeezing the handles together will cause the crown to be elevated, but care must be taken to prevent damage to fine, fragile margins, especially on porcelain crowns.

The Easy Pneumatic Crown and Bridge Remover - creates impact from compressed air.

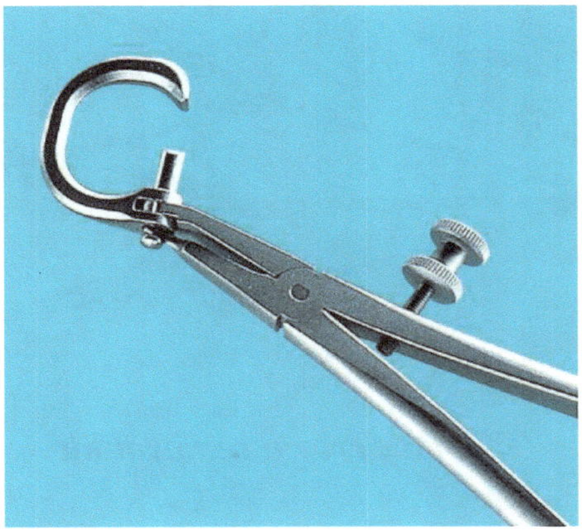

Kavo pneumatic crown remover

Another interesting technique designed to remove a crown without causing damage is performed using the Richwil Crown and Bridge Remover. This material is a water-soluble resin that is softened using warm water. The small block of material is placed on the crown to be removed, and the patient bites into this material until the resin cools and hardens, at which point the patient opens his/her mouth, generating enough force to pull the crown off. Care must be taken by the clinician to refrain from using this technique when the opposing tooth is extensively restored because the opposing restoration may inadvertently be removed during the procedure.

K pliers (GC) - uses small replaceable rubber tips and emery tips to enable a firm grasp of the crown without damaging it.

Other instruments of this kind are-

- Wynman crown gripper (Miltex)
- The Trial crown remover
- The Trident crown placer/ remover

Justman and Krell [JOE 1993] described a technique for removing provisionally cemented crowns that can help prevent both crazing of the porcelain and damage to the margin, or aspiration of the crown by the patient. They recommended that the rubber dam be attached to the wings of a clamp and the jaws of the clamp placed coronally to the margin of the restoration. The rubber dam is released from the wings and positioned with the rubber between the jaws of the retainer and the restoration to provide a buffer. The beaks of a Steiglitz forceps can then be placed in the retainer holes, with leverage more safely applied until the restoration is loosened.

Other techniques, such as vibrations, have also been successful.

Recently, Maillefer announced the new WamKey crown removal system. This new system provides the key to a fast, risk-free and painless crown removal. Designed for ease-of-use, the WamKey is inserted into the crown after a small access hole is made using a bur. Turning the key with two fingers and applying minimal force, the crown 'pops' up, minimising the risk of fracture.

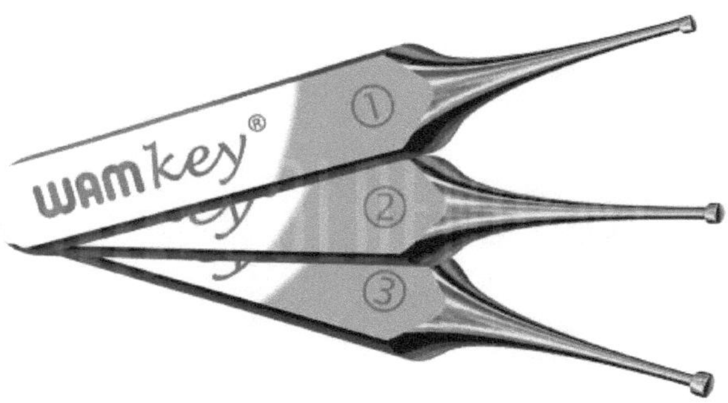

Wamkey crown removal kit

Advantages:

- Designed for simplicity & effectiveness: Reduced risk of fracturing or damaging root/ligament and clinically safe.
- Limited force needed for effective removal: More acceptable procedure. Pain-free for patients.
- Reduced preparation time: Time and cost savings.

- Option to re-use crown (temporarily/permanently): Cost-effective investment that guarantees success.

If the dentist is not able to remove the crown, the following precautions should be taken.

- A fibreoptic system can be used for increased visibility.
- Initial access opening should be done without a rubber dam, to enhance the visualisation of the crown relative to other teeth
- Water spray and high-speed diamond burs should be used. The patient should be warned ahead of time of a possible fracture. The porcelain should be cut in a light shaving manner. Once the porcelain has been penetrated, a sharp carbide bur (transmetal bur) should be used to complete the access preparation.

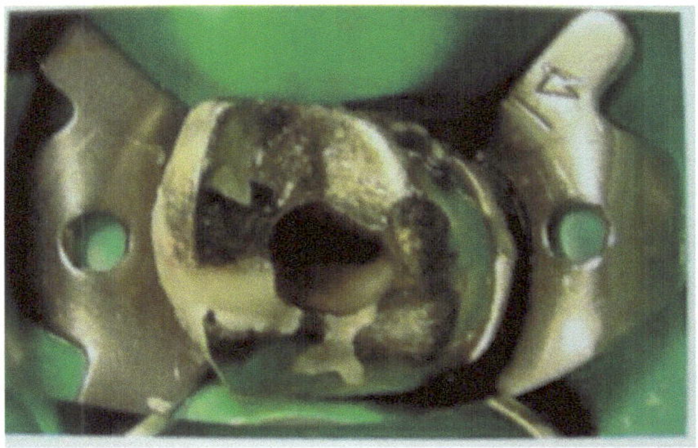

Access opening through the metal crown

- The prepared access cavity should be well irrigated before entering any of the canals. This will help prevent carrying metallic or composite fragments into the canal space.

ACCESS CAVITY PERFORATIONS

A perforation is an undesirable communication between the pulp space and the external tooth surface. It may occur at any level in the chamber or along the length of the root canal. It may occur during preparation of the access cavity, root canal space, or post space.

Access preparations allow the locating, cleaning and shaping of all root canals. In the process of searching for canal orifices, perforations of the crown can occur either peripherally through the sides of the crown or through the floor of the chamber into the furcation.

If the access cavity perforation is above the periodontal attachment, the first sign of the presence of an accidental perforation will often be the presence of leakage, either saliva into the cavity or sodium hypochlorite out into the mouth. At this time, the patient will notice the unpleasant taste.

When the crown is perforated into the periodontal ligament, bleeding into the access cavity is often the first indication of an accidental perforation. To confirm the suspicion of such an unwanted opening, a small file can be placed through the opening and a radiograph taken. The film will clearly demonstrate that the file is not in a canal. In some instances, a perforation may initially be thought to be a canal orifice; placing a file into this opening will provide the necessary information to identify this error. Access cavity perforation occurs when there is

- Failure in orientation of the bur to the long axis of the tooth.
- Failure to complete the convenience form of extension, before the entrance of the shaft of the bur, this usually leads to perforation in the labiocervical region.
- In the maxillary premolars, failure to observe the distal axial inclination of the tooth will result in perforation of the mesiocervical region by-passing the receded pulp.
- Maxillary First Premolar Is The Most Commonly Perforated Tooth.

Perforation of the coronal walls above the alveolar crest can generally be repaired intracoronally without the need for surgical intervention.

Temporary filling material like Cavit will usually serve to seal these types of perforations during endodontic treatment.

Perforations into the periodontal ligament, whether laterally or into the furcation, should be done as soon as possible to minimise the injury to the tooth's supporting tissues. It is also important that the material used in the repair provides a good seal and does not cause further tissue damage.

Several materials have been recommended for perforation repair [(4, 5):] Cavit, amalgam, calcium hydroxide paste, super EBA, glass ionomer cement, gutta-percha, tricalcium phosphate or haemostatic agents such as Gelfoam.

Alhadainy and Abdalla[6] (JOE 1998) did an in vitro dye penetration study creating an artificial floor using either calcium sulfate or hydroxyapatite and then repairing the perforation with Vitrebond (3M ESPE.). The results indicated that calcium sulfate and hydroxyapatite, used as barriers, significantly improved the sealing ability of Vitrebond and provided successful barriers against its overextension.

Use of absorbable, hemostatic collagen products, such as Collastat OBP and collacote act as an artificial barrier against which the repair material can be condensed.

In recent times, MTA / mineral trioxide aggregate (Pro- Root, Dentsply/Tulsa Dental), a material approved by the US Food and Drug Administration, has shown convincing results, and several studies have supported its use for perforation repairs.

Before the repair of a perforation, it is important to control bleeding, both to evaluate the size and locations of the perforation and to allow placement of the repair material. Calcium hydroxide[7] placed in the area of perforation and left for at least a few days, will leave the area dry and allow inspection of the perforation. Mineral trioxide aggregate[8, 9, 10, 11] in contrast to all other repair materials, may be placed in the presence of blood since it requires moisture to set. It is nevertheless preferable to control bleeding before repair so that the location can be more accurately determined.

The prognosis for a perforated tooth is generally downgraded. The clinical decision is based on the circumstances, such as the perforation size and the existing periodontal condition. Sinai proposed that the prognosis for a tooth with a perforation depends on the location of the perforation, the length of time the perforation is open to contamination, the ability to seal the perforation and accessibility to the main canal. Generally, it can be said that the sooner the repair is undertaken, the better the chance of success. Surgical corrections may be necessary in refractory cases.

Thorough examination of diagnostic preoperative radiographs is the paramount step to avoid this error. Checking the long axis of the tooth and aligning the long axis of the access bur with the long axis of the tooth can prevent unfortunate perforations of a tipped tooth. The presence of location and degree of calcification of the pulp chamber noted on the preoperative radiograph is also important information to use in planning the access preparation. Perforations can also often be associated with inadequate access preparation. Prevention of procedural errors is best accomplished by close attention to the principles of access cavity preparation: adequate size and correct location, both permitting direct access to the root canals. A thorough knowledge of tooth anatomy, specifically pulpal anatomy, is essential for anyone performing root canal therapy.

CROWN FRACTURES

Crown fractures of teeth undergoing root canal therapy are complications that can be avoided in many instances. The tooth may have a preexisting infraction that becomes a true fracture when the patient chews on the tooth, weakened additionally by an access preparation.

Recognition of such fractures is usually by direct observation. Infractions are often recognised first after the removal of existing restoration in preparation for the access. When infractions become true fractures, parts of the crown may be mobile.

Crown fractures usually have to be treated by extraction unless the fracture is of a chisel type, in which only the cusp or part of the crown is involved. In such cases, the loose segment can be removed, and treatment can be completed. If the fracture is more extensive, the tooth may not be restorable and needs to be extracted. Crowns with infractions should be supported with circumferential bands or temporary crowns during endodontic treatment.[1]

Prognosis for a tooth with a crown fracture, if it can be treated at all, is likely to be less favourable than for an intact tooth, and the outcome is unpredictable. Crown infractions may spread to the roots, leading to vertical root fractures.

Prevention is simple. The occlusion should be reduced before the working length is established. In addition to preventing this error, it will also aid in reducing discomfort following endodontic therapy.

INSTRUMENTATION ERRORS

Instrumentation errors are commonly associated with excessive and inappropriate dentin removal during the cleaning and shaping phase of endodontics. Most of the procedural errors are related to over-instrumentation.

Excessive canal preparation can weaken the tooth and even fracture the root tip. Roots that have an hourglass configuration in cross-section (e.g., mesial roots of mandibular molars and roots of maxillary premolars) are particularly prone to canal stripping – a term used when root perforations result from excessive flaring during canal preparation. Such flaring can also weaken the tooth. It causes a vertical root fracture to occur during the filling procedure. Over instrumentation can also lead to canal ledgings, apical transportations and perforations.

Gutmann and Dumsha proposed a range of sizes to be used as a guideline for the apical termination of the canal preparation. [2]

Tooth group	Final apical size preparation
Maxillary centrals	35-60
Maxillary laterals	25-40
Maxillary canines	30-50
Maxillary premolars	25-40
Maxillary molars MB/DB	25-40
Maxillary molars palatal	25-50
Mandibular incisors	25-40
Mandibular canines	30-50
Mandibular premolars	30-50
Mandibular molars MB/ML	25-40
Mandibular molars distal	25-50

LEDGE FORMATION

A ledge is an artificially created irregularity on the surface of the root canal that prevents the placement of instruments to the apex of an otherwise patent canal. Occasionally, even skilled and careful clinicians develop canal ledges when treating teeth with unsuspected aberrations in canal anatomy.

Causes of ledge formation[1, 2]

1. Ledges are formed in the root canal mainly due to failure in establishing proper access activity that allows direct access to the apical part of the canals.
2. Ledges are also formed from using straight or too large steel instruments in a curved canal.
3. During instrumentation, failing to gradually increase the size of the file when enlarging the canal. (Failure to use the files in sequential order).
4. Attempt to retrieve broken instruments or filling material during endodontic re-treatment.
5. Attempt to prepare the calcified canal.
6. Incidence of ledging is more frequent while doing the reaming technique.

Detection of ledge

1. When the instruments are introduced into the canal after establishing the working length, a ledge will prevent the instrument from reaching its full working length.
2. Loss of tactile sensation at the apical region when the tip passes into the lumen.
3. Feeling of hitting a solid wall.
4. When the ledge is suspected, a radiograph is taken with the instrument in the place of the ledge. This will provide additional information about the ledge formation.

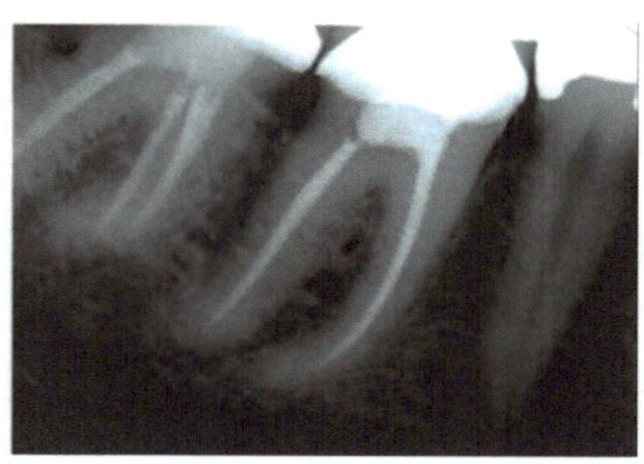

Ledging of all 3 canals in the second molar

Correction of ledge — simplified protocol

- Detect the ledge

- Use a small stainless-steel file (No. 8–10) to locate the ledge and assess canal curvature.
- Place a tear-shaped silicone stop so the pointed side faces the curve to guide the file along the inner curvature.

- Bypass the ledge

- Use a No. 10 or No. 15 K-file to explore the canal with gentle watch-winding and in-and-out motions.
- If you feel resistance, withdraw slightly, rotate the file 30–60°, then try to advance again.
- Maintain light apical pressure and frequent irrigation and lubrication.
- Take a radiograph when the file reaches full working length to confirm position.

- Confirm the glide path and enlarge cautiously

- After bypassing the ledge with No. 15 (or up to No. 20) and confirming patency, enlarge the glide path gradually with sequential files.
- Check the file tip regularly. If the tip straightens, stop continuing; continuing may deepen the ledge and risk perforation.

- Use of greater-taper NiTi (GT) hand files

- Use GT NiTi hand files only after the canal is bypassed, negotiated, and a reliable glide path is established.
- GT files follow the prepared glide path passively; do not force them.
- After using a GT file, recheck with a No. 10 file to confirm the ledge is reduced or removed.

- Irrigation and chemical precautions

- Keep the canal well irrigated and lubricated throughout the procedure.
- Avoid using EDTA aggressively near deep ledges, because chelation can weaken dentin and increase the risk of perforation.

- Safety and prevention

- Never force instruments. Use small, controlled motions.
- Use magnification (loupes or microscope) and radiographs or CBCT when needed.
- If you cannot bypass the ledge or suspect perforation, consider referral or alternative treatment options.

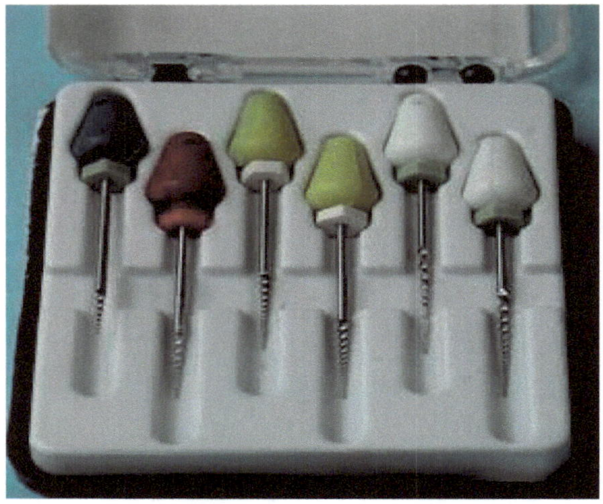

Greater taper files

Prevention of ledge[2]

The outline form of the access cavity should always be prepared in such a way that it does not interfere with the proper instrumentation of the curved canal efficiently, and it should allow an unstrained instrument up to the apical foramen to avoid ledge formation.

Proper convenience form should be achieved for unobstructed filing of curved root canals to prevent ledge formations.

Luebke stated that the entire wall need not be extended in the event of an obstruction occurring due to severely curved root canals; only a portion of the wall obstructing the instruments is modified, giving a clover lip appearance. Hence, he named it as **shamrock preparation**[1]**.**

Proper radiographs should be taken to determine the direction of the root canals and their morphology. Occasionally, when the canal curvature is aligned with the central X-ray beam, the apex appears as a 'bull's-eye' or 'target' image, indicating that the root is sharply curved back on itself. This is a subtle radiographic sign and can be easily overlooked.

Copious irrigation should be used during debridement, cleaning and shaping. Ultrasonics may also assist in the removal of debris.

Instruments must be wiped clean before they are inserted into the canal.

Recapitulation must be used during all instrumentation procedures to ensure an unclogged canal.

Excessive pressure and rotation of instruments inside the canal should be avoided.

Buchanan pointed out the importance of precurving instruments in preparation for curved canals. He recommended the use of pliers in bending instruments.

Yesilsoy, on the other hand, pointed out that using pliers can damage instruments. Finger bending does not produce any damage to the file. However, it will be coated with debris of epithelial cells. Bending of files can be done with rubber gloves or between sterile gauze.

Powell and Simon modified cutting tips to non-cutting tips by grinding the transitional angle from the tip to the first blade. These modified tips maintained the original canal curvature and prevented ledge formations.

The newer instruments with noncutting tips [Flex R files, Flex O files, Flex O reamers] as well as nickel-titanium files have reduced the problem of ledging by allowing the instruments to track the lumen of the canal.

RADICULAR PERFORATIONS

Accidental canal perforations are categorised by location. Radicular perforations can be identified as cervical, mid-root or apical root perforations.

Perforations in all of these locations may be caused by two errors.

(1) Creating a ledge in the canal wall during initial instrumentation and perforation through the side of the root at the point of canal obstruction or root curvature.

(2) Using too large or too long an instrument and either perforating directly through the apical foramen or "wearing" a hole in the lateral surface of the root by over-instrumentation (canal stripping).

CERVICAL CANAL PERFORATIONS

The cervical portion of the canal is most often perforated during the process of locating and widening the canal orifice or inappropriate use of Gates-Glidden burs.

Recognition

- Sudden appearance of blood, which comes from the periodontal ligament. Rinsing and blotting may allow direct visualisation of the perforation; magnification with loupes, an endoscope, or a microscope is very useful in these situations.
- Perforations in the canal can be identified by using paper points. After the canal is dried, if a paper point is introduced into the canal, the perforation site can be identified by observing the blood stain on the paper point.
- If direct visualisation is not adequate to make a definitive identification of a perforation, it may be necessary to place a small file into the area that has been exposed and take a radiograph of the tooth.
- The electronic apex locator is shown to be very valuable in these situations[12].

Correction of the perforation may include both internal and external repair. A small area of perforation may be sealed from inside the tooth. If the perforation is large, it may be necessary to seal first from the inside and then surgically expose the external aspect of the tooth and repair the damaged tooth structure. A material that has been recommended for this is Geristore.

Many materials have been used (amalgam, Cavit, glass ionomer) [4], but the most promising material for almost all types of perforations is MTA. It has been shown to provide a very excellent seal of perforated areas, and since it requires moisture for setting, it is very useful in areas of bleeding.

Prognosis must be considered to be reduced in these types of perforations, and surgical correction may be necessary if a lesion or symptoms develop.

Prevention may be achieved by reviewing each tooth's morphology before entering its pulp space. Additionally, radiographically verifying one's position in the tooth can help prevent perforations before it is too late.

MIDROOT PERFORATIONS

Lateral perforations at the midroot level tend to occur mostly in curved canals, either as a result of

1) Perforating when a ledge has formed during initial instrumentation

2) Along the inside curvature of the root as the canal is straightened out (stripping).

"Stripping" is a lateral perforation caused by over-instrumentation through a thin wall in the root and is most likely to happen on the inside or concave wall of a curved canal, such as the distal wall of the mesial roots in mandibular first molars. Canal stripping results in a fairly long perforation that seriously compromises the outcome of treatment.

Stripping is easily detected by the sudden appearance of haemorrhage in a previously dry canal, if there is tactile resistance of the confines of the canal space, or by a sudden complaint by the patient. A paper point placed in the canal can confirm the presence and location of the perforation.

If any of these occur, it is important to confirm these suspicions radiographically and attempt to correct them before further damage is done. A paper point inserted to the apex will confirm suspected apical perforations.

Successful repair of a lateral perforation depends on the adequacy of the seal established by the repair material. The primary concern is to prevent overextension. So, a resorbable material is first introduced, against which the repair material is condensed to prevent the material from being forced out into the ligament space. If this happens, it will result in a poor seal, despite gentle placement. Castellucci has surmounted this problem, using CollaCote and EBA.

Access to midroot perforation is most often difficult, and repair is not predictable. Calcium hydroxide has been used in the hope of stimulating a biologic barrier against which to pack filling material, but usually, filling material ends up in the perforation area.

Repair of strip perforations has been attempted both non-surgically and surgically. A majority of the techniques propose a two-step method. The root canals are first obturated, and then the defect is repaired surgically.

Allam[13] reported removal of the excess gutta-percha using a hot spatula and cold burnishing the perforation site.

The use of amalgam, gutta-percha, and calcium hydroxide was reported by Biggs et al.[14], and the results using glass ionomer were reported by Goon and Lundergan[15].

All methods have reported limited success, if any. Based on the impressive results using MTA for perforations other than strip perforation, the material might be expected to perform as well as strip perforation repairs also.

Both "stripping" perforation and direct lateral perforation of the root result in a reduction of the prognosis. Loss of tooth structure and integrity of the root wall can lead to subsequent fractures or microleakage owing to the inability to properly seal the perforation. The reduced prognosis must be considered when evaluating the tooth's role in an overall treatment plan.

Berutti and Fedou[16] have shown how delicate the tooth structure is in some areas. In lower first molars at 1.5 mm below the bifurcation, they found the dentin of the root to be 1.2 to 1.3 mm thick from the canal to the cementum. The mesiobuccal canal is in most danger of being stripped.

Peeso wrote about perforated roots, often caused by a rotary instrument, as early as 1903. Modified preparations were formulated to avoid these stripping accidents.

Endodontists at the University of Southern California experienced midroot perforations through their advocacy of Peeso power-driven reamers as an auxiliary aid in enlarging the cervical third of the preparation. To overcome this problem, they developed a new technique. This was termed as **anticurvature filing**. This method stresses the importance of maintaining mesial pressure on the enlarging instruments to avoid the delicate danger zone of the distal wall, where the root is so thin. A similar technique was advocated at Ohio State University. Several other studies reported encouraging results with these methods of filing[17].

Stripping can be prevented by exercising caution in the careful use of rotary instruments inside the canal and following recommendations for canal preparation in curved root canals.

APICAL PERFORATIONS

Perforations in the apical segment of the root canal may be the result of the file not negotiating a curved canal or not establishing accurate working length and instrumenting beyond the apical confines. Perforation of a curved root is the result of ledging, apical transportation, or apical zipping.

Transportation is defined as the removal of the canal wall structure on the outside curve in the apical half of the canal due to the tendency of files to restore themselves to their original linear shape during canal preparation. The term apical zip is also defined as an elliptical shape that may be formed in the apical foramen during preparation of a curved canal when a file extends through the apical foramen and subsequently transports the outer wall.

The maxillary lateral incisor, mesiobuccal and palatal roots of maxillary molars and the mesial root of mandibular molars are most often the sites of these types of perforations, owing to their curvatures.

Apical perforation can also occur in a perfectly straight canal if instrument use exceeds the correct working length. This destroys the resistance form of the root canal preparation at the cementodentinal junction, making it difficult to control the apical extensions of the root canal filling.

An apical perforation should be suspected if the patient suddenly complains of pain during treatment, if the canal becomes flooded with haemorrhage, or if the tactile resistance of the confines of the canal space is lost. If any of these occur, it is important to confirm one's suspicions radiographically and attempt to correct them before further damage is done. A paper point inserted to the apex will confirm a suspected apical perforation.

Efforts to repair an apical perforation may be made in two ways

1. attempting to renegotiate the apical canal segment or
2. Considering the perforation site as the new apical opening and then deciding what treatment the untreated apical root segment will require.

Obturation of both natural and the iatral foramina and of the main body of the canal requires the compacting techniques with heat-softened gutta-percha. Often, surgery is necessary if a lesion is present apically.

If the perforation is caused by overinstrumentation, corrective treatment includes re-establishing tooth length short of the original length and then enlarging the canal, with larger instruments, to that length. A careful adaptation of the primary filling point, often blunted, is essential. The canal is then cautiously filled to that length, so that the resistance form thus created will prevent filling extrusion out of the apex.

Creating an apical barrier is another technique that can be used to prevent overextensions during root canal filling. Materials used include dentin chips, calcium hydroxide powder, Proplast[18], hydroxyapatite and, more recently, MTA. The material that works best in the hands of the individual clinician should be used. The solution is often a compromise but is usually preferable to a surgical correction.

There are more apical perforations than perforations in other areas of the pulp space. Fortunately, with successful repair, apical perforations have less adverse effect on prognosis than more coronal perforations.

MANAGEMENT OF PERFORATIONS

Regardless of the cause, the perforation is an invasion into the supporting tissue that initially incites inflammation and loss of attachment. Ultimately, this may compromise the prognosis of the treatment. An interdisciplinary approach is needed to decide whether to extract or direct efforts towards the non-surgical treatment, surgical correction or both.

NONSURGICAL PERFORATION REPAIR

Factors Influencing Perforation Repair

When evaluating the prognosis of a perforated tooth, several variables must be considered individually and collectively to properly guide treatment.

Four dimensions of a perforation must always be considered, which synergistically affect the treatment outcome.

1) Level
2) Location
3) Size
4) Time

Level

Perforation can occur in the coronal, middle and apical third of the roots. Furcal perforations have similar consideration as the coronal one-third perforations. Perforation at this level threatens the sulcular attachment and poses different treatment challenges than the perforations occurring more apically. In general, the more apical the perforation, the more favourable the prognosis.

Location

Perforations can occur circumferentially on the buccal, lingual, mesial and distal aspects of the roots. The location of the perforation is not so important when the non-surgical treatment is selected. However, its position is critical and may preclude surgical access if this approach is considered.

Size of the perforation

Perforation size greatly affects the establishment of a fluid impervious seal. The area of a circular-shaped perforation can be mathematically described as πr [6]. Therefore, doubling the perforation size with any bur or instrument increases the surface area to seal fourfold.

Time

Regardless of the cause, perforation should be repaired as soon as possible to discourage further loss of the attachment and prevent the sulcular breakdown. Chronic perforation exhibiting loss of sulcular attachment poses treatment challenges that potentially escalate to the surgical correction and efforts directed toward guided tissue regeneration procedures.

The other factors involved are:

Periodontal condition

Teeth that have been perforated must be thoroughly examined periodontally; especially the sulci of the teeth must be carefully probed. If the attachment apparatus is intact without any pocket, timing is critical, and the treatment is ideally directed towards the non-surgical repairing of the defect. However, if there is periodontal breakdown with the resultant loss of attachment, interdisciplinary consultations, including orthodontic, periodontic and endodontic consultations, should guide the treatment planning sequence and prognosis. In these instances, a decision must be made between the nonsurgical repairs and the surgical correction, recognising that, at times, combined treatment may be required to salvage the tooth.

Esthetics

Perforations in the anterior region can definitely affect the esthetics. Patients who exhibit a high lip line can be esthetically compromised by soft- tissue defects such as cleft, recession or discrepancies in the incisogingival dimensions of the crown.

When compared with the adjacent teeth, traditional restoration, when used for the repair, contributes to the tooth discolouration. Tooth colored restoration material should be carefully selected in the areas where esthetically needed.

Vision

Magnification glasses, head lamps and transillumination devices facilitate vision and are important adjuncts in the perforation repair.

The dental operating microscope has dramatically improved the vision, predictability of the non-surgical repair and reduced the need for surgical intervention. Microsurgical approach comes into effect when the area of perforation is inaccessible or when the prognosis for non- surgical repair is poor.

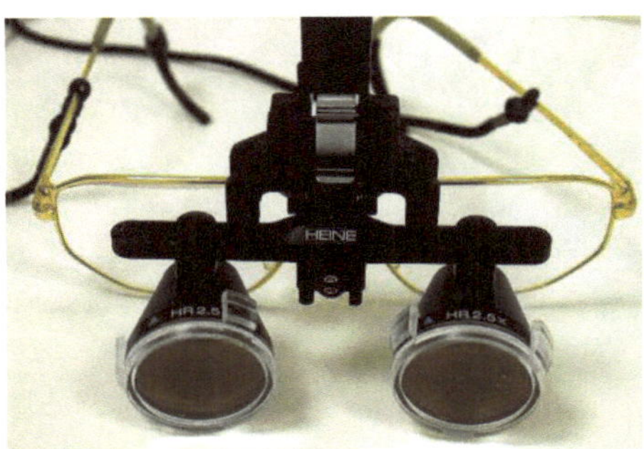

Magnifying loupe

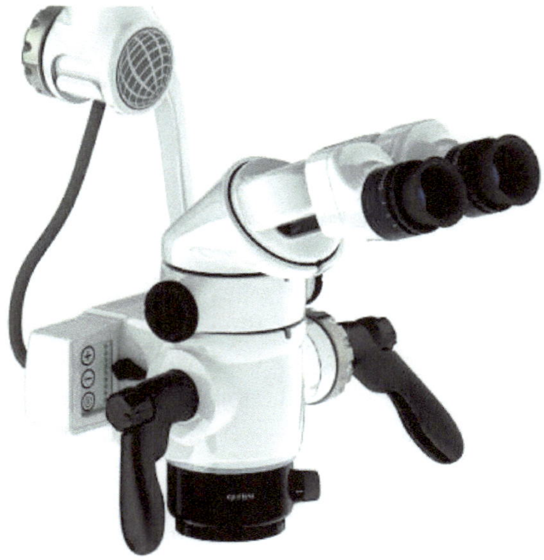

Dental operating microscope

Indications for microsurgery

1. large perforations
2. resorption defects
3. failure of healing after non-surgical repair
4. Large overfills or defects intra coronally

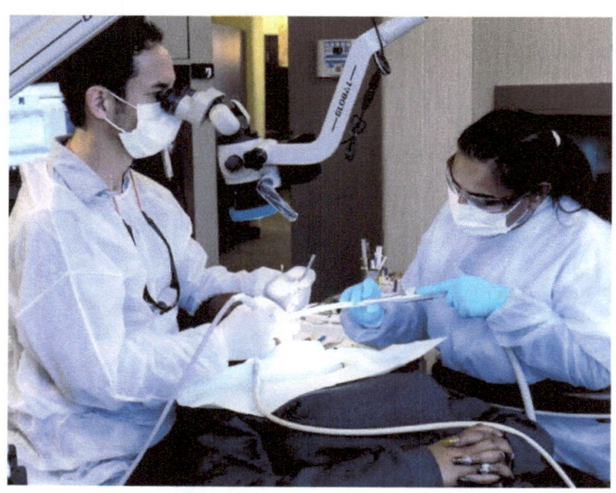

Microsurgery

MATERIALS USED IN PERFORATION REPAIR

1) Hemostatics
2) Barrier material
3) Restoratives

Hemostatics[19]

Perforation defects exhibit massive bleeding. A dry field enhances vision while creating an environment for the predictable placement of a restorative agent.

Calcium hydroxide[5]

Calcium hydroxide is one of the best and time-honoured materials used in dentistry. This material is passively syringed into the canal. It is pushed hydraulically into the defect and allowed to remain in the defect for 4- 5 minutes or longer. The calcium hydroxide is then flushed from the field using sodium hypochlorite solution. Two or three applications of placing and then removing the calcium hydroxide usually begin to control bleeding. If the hemostasis cannot be achieved in such applications, calcium hydroxide is left in the canal until a future appointment.

Collagen[20]

A wide variety of collagen-based hemostatic agents are available for use as local hemostatic material. The principal differences are in the microstructure and the density of the collagen. It acts as a mild allergen, but this can be avoided when highly purified animal collagen is used. Mechanism of action is by stimulation of platelet adhesion, platelet aggregation and activation of factor XII (Hageman factor). A mechanical plug forms at the collagen-blood wound interface. It does not increase the incidence of infection, but it delays early bone repair. Osseous regeneration proceeds without any foreign body reaction. Collagen-based material is very difficult to place because of the tendency to adhere to the wet surface.

Commercially available materials are

- Collocate (Integra Life Sciences, Plainsboro),
- Collostat (American Medical Products Corp)
- Hemocollagene (Ethicon, Pis-cataway)

Surgicel

It is a chemically sterilised material prepared through oxidation of regenerated alpha cellulose (oxycellulose). The basic element of the Surgicel is polyacrylamide, which is spun into threads and then woven into gauze. Surgicel has a pH level of 3. Because of its low pH, it can retard healing. It is primarily a physical hemostatic agent, which acts as a barrier to blood, and as time goes on, it becomes a sticky mass that serves as an artificial coagulum. It does not enhance the clotting mechanism. Resorption of this material is in 120 days.[5]

Gelfoam

- It is a gelatin-based sponge
- It is water-insoluble and biologically resorbable.
- It stimulates the intrinsic pathway of coagulation.
- The initial effect of the gelfoam is a decrease in the rate of healing

Bone wax

- It is 77% bees wax and 12 % isopropyl palmitate.
- Healing of bone is poor
- It produces a chronic inflammatory bone reaction
- It is no longer advised.

Ferric sulphate:

Ferric sulphate produces hemostasis in 5 minutes. It does not affect normal healing. It produces only a mild foreign body reaction. A similar product, MONSEL'S (ferric subsulphate) solution, has been used as a hemostatic agent.

Its usage has been reduced because it produces tissue necrosis for up to 2 weeks. Ferric sulphate is the best hemostatic agent, but it leaves a coagulum that can promote bacterial growth, compromise the seal at the tooth and the restorative interface and affect the prognosis.

Barrier materials

The two main challenges in attempting the perforation repair are hemostasis and the controlled placement of the material in the perforation area. Barrier material, which is placed in the perforation area, will provide a dry field or a back stop to condense the restorative materials against it.

When a barrier membrane is placed over the body defects and closely adapted to the surrounding bone surface, an environment that prevents invasion of competing non-osteogenic cells from the overlying soft tissues can be created. This environment provides the bony defect time to heal.

Guided tissue regeneration

Guided tissue regeneration[21] (GTR) is a procedure used to regenerate lost attachment apparatus through differential tissue response. The objective of GTR in endodontic microsurgery is to enhance the quality and quantity of bone regeneration in the periapical region and to accelerate bone growth in circumscribed bone cavities after endodontic surgery.

Dahlin and colleagues were the first to apply the concept of GTR to bone surgery, creating the guided bone regeneration (GBR) and subsequently applied it to endodontic surgery. Melcher (1976) stated that the cells that repopulate the exposed root surface determine the nature of the attachment that will form.

Several commercially available membranes are currently available.

Non resorbable

- Gortex membrane

It has the disadvantage that it has to be removed during a second follow-up surgical procedure, some six weeks after the initial procedures.

Resorbable

Collagen products

• Biomend

• Bioguide

• Bicon absorbable 100 % synthetic membrane

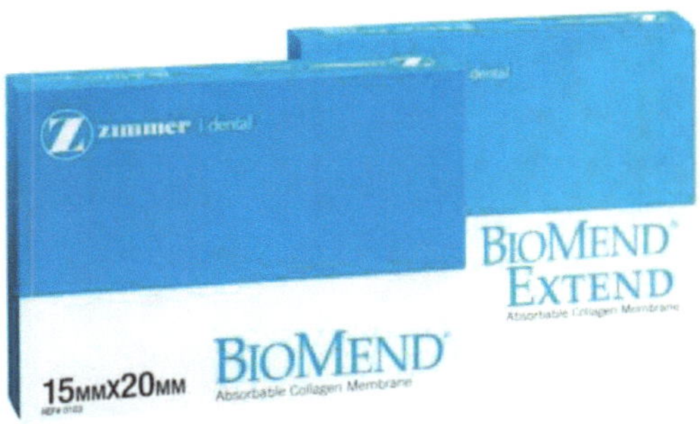

Biomend collagen

Polylactic acid

• Resolute adapt

Regenerative materials that support the membrane

Bone graft materials have two main functions[22].

• Act as a mechanical substructure that supports the membrane and the overlying soft tissues

• To serve as a biologic component that enhances bone formation.

Bone graft material can be categorised as osteoconductive or osteoinductive.

An osteoconductive material provides a framework into which bone can grow. The material is gradually absorbed and remodelled.

An osteoinductive material stimulates the production of new cells such that healing occurs more quickly.

Types of bone grafts

Autogenous graft - Ramus, chin, iliac crest

Allograft - Demineralised freeze-dried human bone.

(e.g.) Osteofil, Dynagraft

Xenograft - Inorganic bovine / porcine bone particles

(e.g.) Bio oss, Osteograft

Ceramic/synthetic grafts - Calcium sulfate, Calcium phosphate, Hydroxyapatite

(e.g.) Perioglas, Osteoset, Biogran.

Bioactive proteins - Bone morphogenic protein (Experimental)

Combination graft - Allograft, Xenograft or Ceramic / Synthetic graft and bioactive protein, Pepgen P 15

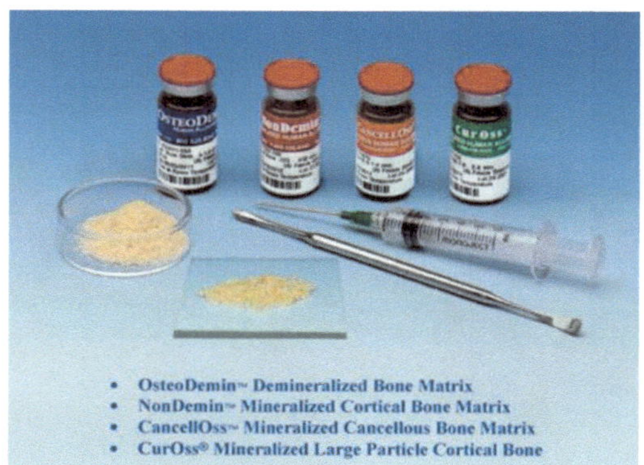

Bonegraft materials

Points to remember while using the barrier membrane are

1. The membrane should extend at least 2-3 mm beyond the margins of the bone cavity.
2. A secluded space must be created underneath the membrane to allow the growth of new tissue
3. The membrane should be totally submerged because an exposed membrane increases the risk of infection.
4. The membrane must be stable and immovable
5. The membrane must act as a selective barrier for at least 6-8 weeks.
6. Mobile teeth must be splinted
7. A strict oral hygiene regimen must be followed.

In general, barrier material can be divided into resorbable and non-resorbable barrier materials. However, sometimes the restorative material will dictate the barrier that is selected.

Resorbable barrier material

Once the internal bleeding in the tooth is managed, the resorbable material is placed into the perforation defect nonsurgically, and no material should be left inside the tooth structure. The resorbable material should be confined to the bone. The barrier should conform to the anatomy of the furcation area or the root surface involved. Although there are several materials available, collagen and calcium sulphate materials are the best choice because of their better handling.

Collagen

Based on the defect and the available access, Collacote is cut to appropriate sizes and carried into the access cavity. The material is placed incrementally through the tooth and into the osseous defect until the solid barrier corresponding to the cavosurface of the root surface is established. Hemostasis is achieved in 2 to 5 minutes. Collagen is used in conjunction with the amalgam, Super EBA and other non-bonded restorative materials. Collagen is not indicated in adhesive dentistry because its moisture will contaminate the restorative materials.

Calcium sulphate

It has been used as a substitute for bone graft to fill the bone defects since the late 1800s.

The presence of calcium sulphate in the bone wound does not inhibit bone formation. It is gradually removed from the wound. Deposition of cementum and osseous healing proceed normally. As a hemostatic agent, it acts as a physical barrier.

Calcium sulfate rapidly sets as brick-hard, and it is easily finished with ultrasonic finishing instruments (UFI). The ultrasonic finishing systems are able to work deep within the root canal space. Their port technologies dispense the irrigants into the field of operation. Calcium sulphate is the choice of material when using the principles of wet bonding. The perforation defect can be rinsed of contaminants and prepared for adhesion dentistry.

Nonresorbable barrier materials:

Mineral Trioxide Aggregate[8, 23, 24,9,10,11]

Mineral trioxide aggregate (MTA), based on Portland cement, was developed by Torabinejad in 1993. It has many clinical applications and represents an extraordinary breakthrough for the management of radicular repair. MTA has excellent tissue-bio-compatible properties. It is used as a nonresorbable barrier and restorative material. It is the material of choice when there is a chance of moisture contamination. It can be used as the barrier material on which other material can be packed.

Constituents:

- Calcium oxide 50-75 %
- Silicon dioxide 15-25%
- Bismuth oxide for radio opacity

When blended, these raw materials produce Tricalcium silicate, dicalcium silicate, Tricalcium aluminates and tetra calcium alumino ferrite. On addition of water, the cement hydrates to form a silicate hydrate gel, which hardens in about 3 hours.

Viscosity-enhanced root end filling material (VEREFM)

• It is a new material formulated using Portland cement as a base material.

• Bismuth and other components are added to improve the radiopacity and handling characteristics.

Restorative materials:

Success in repairing the perforations is to select a material that is easy to use, which is non-resorbable, biocompatible, esthetically pleasing, and that provides a complete seal.

Amalgam

Rhein in 1897 used amalgam [4, 5, 25] to seal the pulp canal after complete root resection. Initially, copper amalgam was used, and later silver amalgam was used widely.

Disadvantages:

- The placement of amalgam as a restorative of choice in a perforated root, which has a metallic post or crown for restoration, could create a galvanic couple and generate a significant amount of galvanic current. Sufficient depth must be provided to place base material such as calcium hydroxide or zinc oxide eugenol to prevent galvanism.
- Amalgam may be scattered in the perforated area and may cause staining.

Zinc oxide eugenol.

Zinc oxide eugenol is a very old material, used since the 1870s. It has many disadvantages. Eugenol is released from ZOE mixtures, which can be irritating to the surrounding tissue. When ZOE comes into contact with water, it undergoes surface hydrolysis, producing zinc hydroxide and eugenol. Other materials have been added to the basic ZOE mixture in an effort to increase the strength and radioopacity and reduce the solubility of the final material (IRM, Super-EBA).

Super EBA resin cement:

Coleman and Kirk, in 1965, first recommended the use of EBA as root end filling material. It is a non-reabsorbable material. It comes in powder and liquid form.

Powder –

- 60% zinc oxide eugenol
- 6% natural resin
- 34% Aluminium oxide

Liquid –

- 62.5% ethoxybenoic acid
- 37.5 % eugenol.

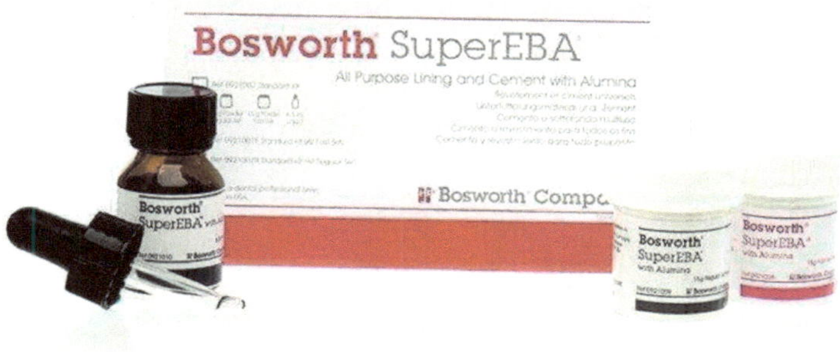

EBA is available in two forms- fast set and regular set. It has adequate working time, and it does not need any cavity preparation. Its radiopacity and sealing ability are similar to IRM. It is less leaky than amalgam. The environment of the super EBA may affect its long-term stability, which has been shown to disintegrate over time in acid environment[26,25]. Biologically, it is well tolerated.

Super EBA has a limited antibacterial effect. Its cytotoxicity is similar to that of amalgam and IRM.

<u>Intermediate restorative material (IRM)</u>

Powder contains more than 75% zinc oxide and approximately 20% polymethacrylate. Liquid contains greater than 99% eugenol and less than 1% acetic acid. It seals better than amalgam, and it is not affected by root end conditioning agents. It has good tissue tolerance[27]. It does not have any hard tissue-forming capacity.

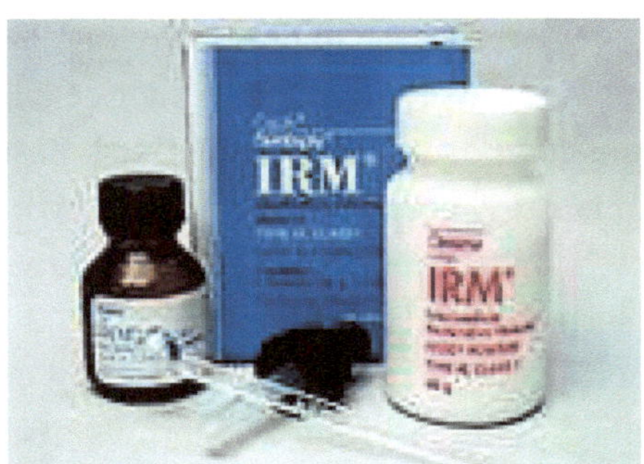

IRM material

Glass ionomer[4].

It consists of polyacrylic acid and a glass powder such as aluminosilicate. Glassionomer cements can be either light or chemical cure. Seal and marginal adaptation of the light cure is superior to the chemical cure. Seal is better than amalgam and similar to that of IRM. Glassionomer cements are susceptible to attack by moisture during the initial setting period, resulting in increased solubility and decreased bond strength. The cytotoxicity does not differ from IRM and super EBA or amalgam.

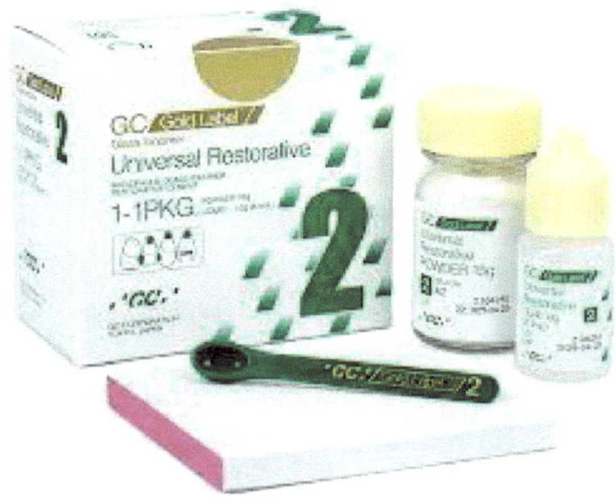

Glass ionomer cement

Composite resin restorations.

Composite resin material has some desirable properties[28] and it can be considered as a repair material. They have good sealability. They leak less than amalgam. Moisture and blood contamination reduce bond strength and increase leakage.

(e.g.)

- Retroplast [Retroplast trading]

Retroplast[29]

It is a dentin bonding composite resin system developed in 1984. The formulation was changed in 1990, when silver was added in place of ytterbium trifluoride and ferric oxide. It comes as a two-part form that forms a dual-cure composite resin when mixed. Paste A is composed of Bis – GMA / TEGDMA in the ratio of 1:1, benzoyl peroxide, N, N-di-(2- hydroxyethyl) p-toluidine, and BHT. Paste B consists of a resin ytterbium trifluorideaerosil ferric oxide. A Gluma-based bonding agent is used to adhere to the root surface. Working time is 1-1/2 to 2 minutes. It is well tolerated and promotes a good healing response. Healing shows deposition of cementum in the root surface and regeneration of periodontium, including insertion of Sharpy's fibers[30].

Resin Ionomer Suspension.

Geristore (Dentsply Tulsa dental) & Dyract (Denmat corporation)

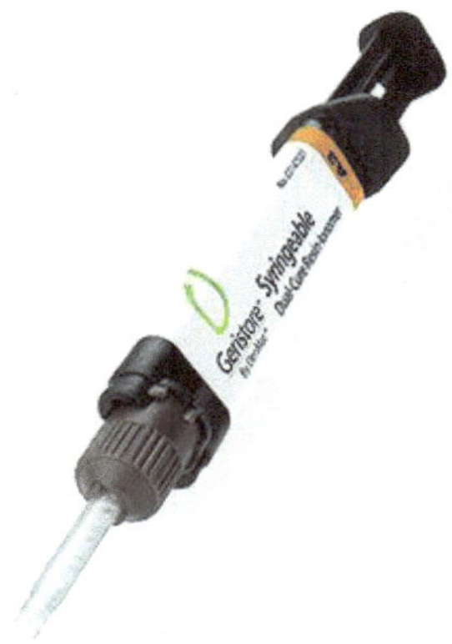

Geristore

It is a combination of resin and glass ionomer, combining various properties of both materials. These materials require light activation and resin-dentin bonding agents to attach to the root surface. Geristore is recommended as a repair material for subgingival defects and iatrogenic perforations. It is used as an adjunct to GTR. Geristore's dual curing paste/ paste formulation is a hydrophilic Bis-GMA with a long-term fluoride release. Light activation is for 40 seconds and cures the material to a depth of 4mm. In vitro leakage studies of Geristore and Dyract indicate that these materials leak less than IRM, amalgam or super EBA. Geristore has the leakage pattern of MTA.

These materials are more sensitive to moisture than conventional glass-ionomer cements. A dry environment produces strong bonds. Geristore has the potential to regenerate periradicular tissues. Histological evidence of cellular attachment is seen.

Mineral trioxide aggregate[8, 24,9,10,11]

When MTA powder is mixed with water, hydration takes place.

Hydration of the powder produces a colloidal gel that solidifies into a hard structure consisting of discrete crystals in an amorphous matrix. The crystals are composed of calcium oxide, and the amorphous region is composed of 33% calcium, 49% phosphate, 2% carbon, 3% chloride and 6% silica.

MTA has the longest setting time of 2 hours and 45 minutes. Compressive strength is lowest at 24 hours-40 MPa, but it increases to 67MPa, 21 days after mixing. The compressive strength, radiopacity and the solubility of MTA are those of amalgam, super EBA and IRM. But it is more radiopaque than IRM and super EBA. Initially, the pH is 10.2, which rises to 2.5, three hours after mixing; pH is about 9.5 at 168 hours after mixing. Mean particle size is 10μm. The range of particle size is from 0.1 µm to 100 µm. Holland et al. theorised that the tricalcium oxide in MTA reacts with tissue fluid to form calcium hydroxide, resulting in hard tissue formation. Studies in dogs have reported less periradicular inflammation and cementum deposition immediately adjacent to the material.

Augmentation of new cementum is necessary to make the apical barrier more resistant to the penetration of microorganisms —a biological barrier. Scanning electron microscopic analysis indicated that cementoblasts could reattach and grow on MTA. In addition, a strong expression of the osteocalcin gene was seen after application of MTA. MTA also increases the production of both proinflammatory and anti-inflammatory cytokines from osteoblasts.

<u>White MTA</u>

This material is a variance from its original formula. It is white in colour.

The chemical formula is similar to the original formula, except for the omission of the alumino ferrite phase. Radiopacity is equal for both formulas.

Techniques for non-surgical repair

The specific barrier and the restorative material selected to repair the perforation site should be based on sound research, judgment, experience, training, esthetics, ease in handling and the advantages and disadvantages of a particular material in a specific clinical setting.

Treatment Sequence for Root Perforation Repair

1. Diagnose the perforation - Identify the perforation clinically and radiographically. Look for root filling or restorative material extending beyond the confines of the root canal.
2. Confirm location - Take angled radiographs to determine the exact location and surface of the root affected by the perforation.
3. Periodontal assessment - Perform a thorough periodontal examination, especially for cervical and mid-root perforations, as these are often associated with epithelial down-growth.
4. Prepare the canal - If the canal is not adequately shaped, enlarge and prepare it to improve access, enhance visualisation of the defect, and minimise instrumentation after repair.
5. Repair the perforation first - Repair the perforation before completing root canal treatment to control bleeding, confine irrigants, and achieve an effective seal.
6. Maintain canal patency - Preserve the physiological canal pathway by placing a gutta-percha point, cotton pellet, or collagen plug apical to the perforation to prevent blockage during repair.
7. Place repair material - Mineral Trioxide Aggregate (MTA) is the material of choice because it provides an excellent seal, sets in the presence of blood, and promotes cementum-like tissue formation.

8. Complete endodontic treatment - After successful perforation repair and adequate setting of the repair material, proceed with cleaning, shaping, obturation, and final restoration.

Advantages and Disadvantages of MTA

Advantages	Disadvantage
Excellent sealing ability	Long setting time
Sets even in the presence of blood or moisture	Not ideal for gingival (cervical) perforations requiring immediate restoration
Biocompatible	
Promotes cementum-like tissue formation and periodontal healing	
High success rate for perforation repair	

Steps in Perforation Repair

1. **Prepare coronal access** to expose the perforation site.
2. **Locate the root canals** and perform preliminary instrumentation to create enough space and prevent blockage by the repair material.
3. **Clean the perforation area** by removing contaminated dentin using ultrasonic tips or Gates-Glidden drills.
4. **Irrigate the perforation**:
    - Use **sodium hypochlorite** for small perforations.
    - Use **normal saline** for large perforations.
    - Avoid pushing the irrigating solution beyond the perforation.
5. **Control bleeding (hemostasis)** using **collagen, calcium sulphate, or calcium hydroxide**.
    - **Do not use ferric sulphate**, as it may compromise the seal and promote bacterial growth.
6. **Protect the root canal** by placing a **gutta-percha point, paper point, or collagen** into the canal to prevent blockage by the repair material.
    - Avoid using a severed file because it is difficult to remove.
7. **Assess the need for an external matrix**.
    - If the surrounding bone supports the defect, a matrix is not required.
    - If there is a large bony defect, place an external matrix.

8. **Place the external matrix (if required)** using collagen, freeze-dried demineralised bone allograft (FDDB), hydroxyapatite, Gelfoam, or calcium sulphate.
    - Do not condense the matrix forcefully to avoid damage to nearby structures.
9. **Place the repair material (MTA)** into the perforation using a small syringe, amalgam carrier, or paper point, and condense it with pluggers or micropluggers.
10. **Place a moist cotton pellet** over the MTA and temporarily seal the tooth to allow the material to set.
11. **Complete the root canal treatment** after the MTA has set, taking care not to disturb the repaired perforation during canal preparation and obturation.

Key Points

- **Material of choice: Mineral Trioxide Aggregate (MTA)**
- **Small perforation:** Irrigate with sodium hypochlorite.
- **Large perforation:** Irrigate with normal saline.
- **Avoid ferric sulfate** for hemostasis.
- **Maintain canal patency** throughout the procedure.

MANAGEMENT OF THE CORONAL ONE-THIRD AND THE FURCAL PERFORATIONS:

The major difference between the coronal one-third and the furcal floor perforations is the shape of the resultant root defect. Mechanical perforations in the furcal floor are generally round, whereas those occurring in the lateral aspect of roots are ovoid by nature in nature.

When managing perforations, the first step is to isolate the perforation site. If the perforation is mechanical and has just occurred, it is probably clean and aseptic. In this situation, if the hemostasis can be accomplished, it can be repaired immediately. If the perforation is chronic and exhibits microleakage, it needs to be cleaned and prepared before receiving the material.

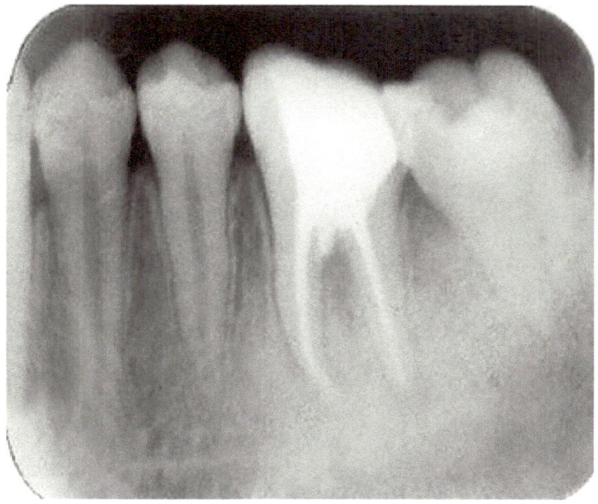

Repaired furcal perforation(MTA)

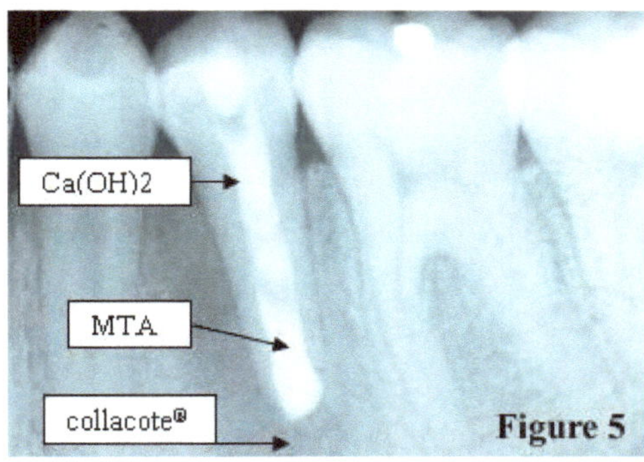

Perforation repair (MTA & collacote)

Ultrasonic finishing instruments are ideal for preparing the perforation site because of their coatings and the irrigation port technologies. Once the area is properly cleaned and prepared, an appropriate barrier material and the restorative material are selected based on the esthetic consideration.

In the coronal one-third of the preparation where esthetics is a main concern, a calcium sulphate barrier in conjunction with adhesion dentistry is the choice. Presently, white MTA is becoming the barrier and the restorative material of choice for repairing esthetic, coronal one-third defects. When esthetics is not a concern, amalgam and super EBA, and more recently grey MTA have been used to repair the coronal one-third perforations.

MANAGEMENT OF PERFORATION IN THE MIDDLE ONE THIRD OF THE ROOT

Iatrogenic perforation in the middle one-third of the root is generally caused by endodontic files, GG drills or a large or misdirected post. By the nature of occurrence, these defects are oval in shape and typically represent a relatively large surface area to seal. In the multirooted tooth, perforation in the furcal area is termed a furcal strip. Middle third perforations have the same technical consideration as the coronal third perforation, except that the defect is located deeper and further away from the access cavity. The factors that must be addressed successfully are hemostasis, access, use of micro instrumentation techniques and selection of the best material in the challenging situation. When managing deeper defects in the lateral walls of the canals, vision is enhanced when direct access is created safely.

In some cases, direct access may not be possible without irreversibly compromising the structural integrity of the tooth. Perforations due to over-instrumentation are sterile, and usually it does not need any micro-instrumentation procedures. Failing endodontic cases that are associated with microleakage may require ultrasonic finishing to clean and to refine the defect in preparation for repair.

In case of large defects, if there is a chance of moisture contamination, it should be repaired first before the three-dimensional obturation of the canal. It is best to prepare the canal minimally before repair; this will facilitate access to the defect and minimize post repair instrumentation.

To prevent obstruction of the root canal space, easily retrievable material is placed in the canal and apical to the defect before the perforation is repaired. Since there is technical difficulty in the access, limited visibility and uncertain moisture-free environment, MTA is the material of choice for both as a barrier and restorative material.

MANAGEMENT OF PERFORATION IN THE APICAL ONE-THIRD

Apical one-third perforations usually occur during the cleaning and shaping procedure. Blocks and ledges invite deep perforation and result from inadequate irrigation and instrumentation, and failure to maintain patency. Recognising the exact cause of the perforation has led to surgical correction using apicoectomy and retrograde filling. In general, it is best to attempt nonsurgical retreatment to enhance the existing restoration.

MTA is the material of choice for repairing deep perforation, especially when a dry environment and technical access are not possible. To prevent the holding file from being frozen in a sea of MTA as it hardens, the instrument is grasped with Steiglitz pliers and moved up and down in 1-2mm amplitude strokes. A radiograph should be taken to confirm the position of MTA and the quality of repair. A wet cotton pellet is placed in the pulp chamber against the MTA, and the patient is dismissed. Upon reentry, the holding file is removed, if the MTA is brick hard, the canal is irrigated, and the final preparation is done gently. Master cone X-ray is taken, and the canal is obturated. It is best to do a follow-up periodically before placing the final restoration.

Even though the best technologies and skills are used, sometimes perforation repair requires surgical treatment.

SURGICAL PERFORATION REPAIR

Surgical management of perforation depends on access to the defect and the relationship to the crestal bone and epithelial attachment. Radicular perforations occurring in the apical one-third pose little problem in management and are amenable to the root end resection technique. Perforation defects in the mesial, distal or buccal can be more easily visualised than the lingual or palatal aspect.

Common causes of mid root perforation include post space preparation and excessive penetration with the rotary intracanal drill or reamers. Accessibility to these areas makes them easier to repair, and if necessary, additional bone can be removed. If the canal is already obturated, any soft tissue, if present, is curetted from the defect and all rough areas are removed. If the canal is not obturated, a GP point is placed in the canal, and the reparative material is packed against it. This prevents canal blockage and, in addition, provides a firm matrix for condensation.

Mid root perforations during post space preparation, which have the post penetrating the periradicular tissue, pose a different problem. If the post is not cemented, perforation is repaired first, and the length of the post is reduced before cementation if the aberrant channel is used for post placement.

If the post has reached beyond the root surface, it must be carefully ground and countersunk into the tooth with a diamond or carbide bur. Good isolation and finger rest are essential to minimise adverse incidents like slipping of the bur and damaging the adjacent tooth structure. Cutting of metal will cause scattering of foreign particles into the adjacent bone.

Surgical manipulation of the mesial or distal perforation is always more difficult because access is limited by root anatomy, position of the defect and the proximity of adjacent root structure. When the perforation is adjacent to the buccal root wall, the cavity is extended buccally to enhance surgical access.

If the perforation is located more lingually or palatally, extension of the proximal root wall may be considered. Lingual perforation is very difficult to repair in the mandibular teeth due to limited surgical access. Surgical access to the maxillary teeth on the palatal aspect is somewhat better.

The development of a periodontal defect is always a potential sequel of the surgical management of mid-root perforation. The proper repositioning and suturing of the reflected tissue is essential in the reestablishment of sound investing periodontium.

Factors considered relative to treatment and prognosis.

- The amount of remaining bone.
- Extent of osseous lesion
- Length of time the defect has been present.
- Presence or absence of periodontal lesion.
- The health of over lying soft tissue.
- Patient oral hygiene.

Perforations in the coronal third of the root are amenable to surgical procedures. When the defect communicates with the gingival sulcus, management of the defect would result in loss of crestal bone or the creation of a potential periodontal pocket. Apically repositioning the flap can be considered to enhance both the position of the defect and the ultimate periodontal and restorative aspects of the tooth.

When cervical perforation is located just apical to the intact epithelium attachment and above the crest, maintenance of the attachment is very difficult and minor soft tissue adjustment is necessary. When a defect is located at the osseous crest, a full-thickness mucoperiosteal flap is reflected, and the defect is cleaned and restored with filling material.

ORTHODONTIC TOOTH EXTRUSION

Orthodontic extrusion is indicated when a perforation defect is present below the crestal bone. However, the desired results cannot be achieved without doing additional crown lengthening. This is necessary to compensate for the coronal movement of the gingival attachment and the alveolar bone, which occur during tooth eruption, resulting in unacceptable esthetics.

In determining the stability of the perforated root for extrusion, the final root crown ratio must be estimated. If the crown is perforated completely below the crestal bone, the postoperative root length will be at least 3mm less than the overall root length because of allowance for 1mm of clinical crown and 2mm of gingival sulcus. Most of the traumatic perforations tend to be oblique rather than horizontal in position. The defect is measured with the periodontal probe to determine the deepest apical extension. The effective root lengthening will begin below this level.

Root lengthening and extrusion will result in unacceptable short roots. They may require splinting.

ROOT RESECTION PROCEDURE:

In 1884, Farrar reported success in root resection procedures. When perforations cannot be treated by any other procedure, sectioning of the tooth is indicated. However, the procedure depends on the periodontal condition.

Technique of root resection procedure:

Root resection on the mandibular or maxillary multirooted tooth implies an angle cut to remove the root from the apex. Flap is reflected. Bone around the root to be resected is removed in a brush stroke manner with a surgical length round bur or fissure bur with a round-ended tip. Removal of furcation bone is also necessary to identify the root anatomy where it joins with the root. Black suggested the removal of the root as close to its furcation. Finally, the surface of the amputated tooth is smoothed.

Two surgical techniques have been advocated in the resection of the root.

1. The first technique is cutting the root directly with a tapered fissure bur at the neck of the tooth, followed by contouring the root surface. Resecting the tooth in this manner will leave a deep trough between the crown and oral mucosa, which serves as a trap for debris.

2. The second technique advocates presurgical crown contouring, in which the portion of the crown over the root to be resected is trimmed away to enhance access to the root to be resected and to reduce the occlusal table over the resected portion of the tooth. In the process of crown alteration, the bur actually begins to cut into the root to be removed at its juncture with the crown, thereby establishing a proper contour from the crown to the furcation.

Surgical length burs are recommended for root resections, especially during resection of wide buccal-lingual roots and during crown contouring.

Before root resection, it is advisable to fill the pulp chamber and coronal third of the root with amalgam or any other root filling material. This will enable the achievement of an immediate seal on the resected root surface and an anatomic marker of the centre portion of the root during resection.

INTENTIONAL REPLANTATION

In 1966, Dr Louis L. Grossman defined replantation as the purposeful removal of a tooth and its almost immediate replacement with the object of obturating the canal apically out of its socket.

Replantation techniques in the past usually failed, with the tooth undergoing varying degrees of resorption. The modern implantation technique, based on biological concepts and the importance of maintaining viability of the periodontal ligament, has led to varying degrees of success.

Indications

Difficult access

Mandibular second molars, where the surgical approach is extremely difficult because of lingually inclined roots and the wide external oblique ridge.

Anatomical limitations

Mandibular bicuspids due to the closeness of the roots to the mental foramen

Perforation in inaccessible areas

Perforations on the buccal surface of the palatal root of maxillary molars, maxillary bicuspids, where surgical repair would result in loss of health of the buccal bone to gain access to the buccal roots

Failed retreatment

Where conventional endodontic therapy, endodontic retreatment and apical surgery are unsuccessful, replantation is the only alternative to extraction.

Patient limitations

Medically compromised and geriatric patients

Contraindications

- Dilacerated roots
- Periodontally compromised roots.
- Teeth with flared roots
- Moderately curved roots and presence of periodontal problems.
- Prognosis is generally good in the case of incisors.

Procedure:

All the necessary materials should be kept ready before extracting the tooth. The tooth should be extracted carefully with minimum trauma to the tooth and to the socket. Elevators should not be used while extracting. Root surface should not be engaged with forceps. After extraction, the root surface must be kept moist by wrapping the root with gauze soaked in a physiological solution, such as Hank's balanced salt solution. Perforation repair is done. The tooth is replanted, and the buccal bone is compressed. The patient may be instructed to bite on a cotton roll or other semisolid material to position the tooth properly in the socket.

Occlusal adjustment is done to minimise traumatic forces on the tooth during the initial stage of healing. A splint may be applied. Patient is instructed to eat a soft diet and avoid sticky foods like candy and chewing gum for at least 7 to 10 days.

TRANSPORTATIONS

Transportation is defined as moving the position of the canal's physiological terminus to a new iatrogenic location on the external root surface.

Foraminal zips or tears are caused by carrying progressively larger and stiffer files to the length.

If the transportation has occurred, the canal exhibits reverse architecture and fails to provide resistance form for the obturating material.

Apical transportation is classified into three types.

Type I (Minor Transportation)

- Minor movement of the apical foramen to a new iatrogenic position.
- Evaluate the amount of remaining dentin before further instrumentation.
- If sufficient dentin is present, create a coronal shape (resistance form) above the new foramen.
- Complete obturation after proper canal shaping.
- Avoid excessive dentin removal, as it may weaken the root or cause strip perforation.

Type II (Moderate Transportation)

- Moderate movement of the apical foramen to a new iatrogenic position.
- The apical one-third of the canal shows greater reverse architecture than Type I.
- Further canal shaping is not recommended because it may further weaken the root.
- Place an apical barrier to control bleeding and provide a stop for obturation.
- Mineral Trioxide Aggregate (MTA) is the material of choice.
- Complete obturation against the MTA barrier.

Type III (Severe Transportation)

- Severe transportation with extensive destruction of the apical canal anatomy.
- The original canal path and apical constriction are completely lost.
- The canal cannot be predictably cleaned, shaped, or obturated through conventional root canal treatment.
- Nonsurgical endodontic treatment has a poor prognosis.
- Periradicular (apical) surgery with root-end resection and retrograde filling is usually the treatment of choice.

- If the tooth is non-restorable or cannot be managed surgically, extraction may be indicated.

Management

Proroot is mixed with anaesthetic solution or sterile water to a heavy, cake-like consistency. A small amount of the material is picked and introduced into the canal with a microtube carrying device, such as a customised spinal tap needle or on the side of a West perforation repair instrument. Proroot is then tamped and coaxed down the canal to approximate length using a customised nonstandard gutta-percha cone as a flexible plugger.

In a straight canal, it can be vibrated with CPR 3, 4 or 5 or moved with an ultrasonic activator instrument. Apical one-third of the canal should be filled with 4-5 mm of MTA, and it should be confirmed radiographically. To ensure moisture, a moist cotton pellet is placed over the MTA and the canal is temporised.

Prevention of perforations and apical transportations

The canal orifice must be located before entering the canal with files. It is most difficult and time-consuming, especially in older patients. An endodontic explorer is the greatest aid in finding the minute orifices by poking action and feeling along the wall of the canal and into the floor of the chamber in the area where the orifices are expected to be.

Bite wing radiographs:

Bitewing radiographs are particularly helpful in estimating the correct depth of penetration and direction of the orifices.

Colour index:

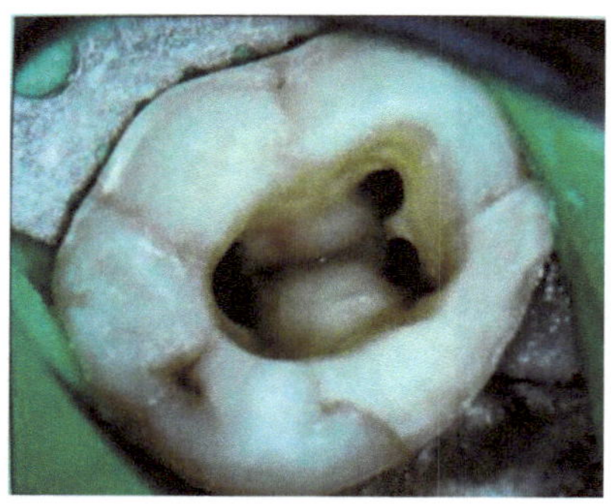

Dentinal map on pulpal floor

Colour is another invaluable aid in finding the canal orifice, especially in molars. The molar triangle is a dark grey or sometimes brown anatomical line present in the pulpal floor. These lines connect the canal orifices. Tracing these lines will lead to one orifice to the second, third or even fourth.

Orifice opener:

Canal orifices are often restrictive, and they need to be flared so that the instruments may enter easily. Orifice openers, from hand-operated to contra-angle powered openers, are helpful.

Gates glidden and the peeso reamers are the most popular instruments in the new instrumentation techniques for both opening of the orifice and deeper penetration of the curved canals. Gates – glidden drills come in sizes 1 to 6, and it is covered under ISO.

Use of a slower hand piece, the Medidenta reduction gear hand piece, the Sensomatic hand piece, the Hitec IMD9GX hand piece, where torque may be controlled as low as 10 rpm, can be used for opening orifices. Lack of tactile sensation is the real problem during the use of engine-driven instruments. However, the use of slow rotaries can improve tactile sensation.

Exploration of the canal

Besides the use of radiographs, the use of a fine curved reamer is a method for determining the curvature of the canals. A curved path finding instrument can be rotated away from a catch or curve on the wall and advanced down the canal to the apical region. This will prevent ledges in the curved canal, which leads to perforations.

While exploring the curved canal with the curved instrument, it is best to search for the unusual curvature towards the direction of the X-rays that is on the buccolingual or in the labio lingual direction, which is not seen in the radiographs, especially in the maxillary molars, lateral incisors and canines. In the mandibular premolars, curvature of the canal toward the buccal or lingual direction is a common occurrence as well.

Termination of the working length:

The length determination procedure determines the apical extent of the instrumentation and the ultimate apical length of the root canal filling. Failure in accurately determining the length of the tooth may lead to apical perforation, which leads to postoperative pain. In addition to this, there is prolonged healing and increased failure due to the incomplete regeneration of cementum, periodontal ligament and the alveolar bone.

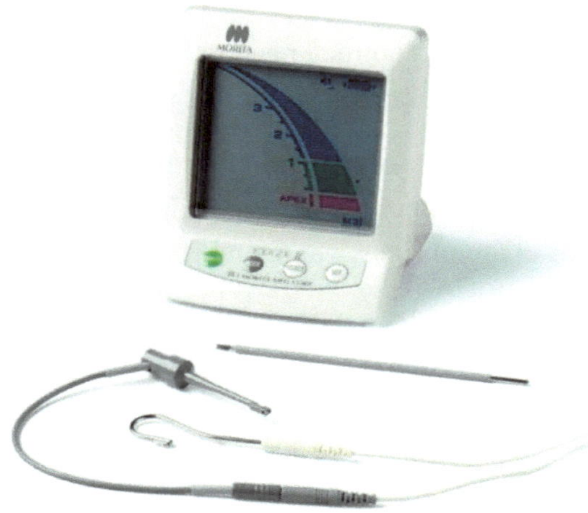

Apex locator

Use of apex locators serves as a useful adjunct for the determination of working length.

Flexible file systems:

Use of a flexible file system in curved canals will prevent ledge formations and perforations.

These files are now being used widely since these instruments have minimised the drastic change in canal path.

1) K- flex

It is a modification of the K-file. Kerr manufacturing company in 1982 introduced K- flex files.

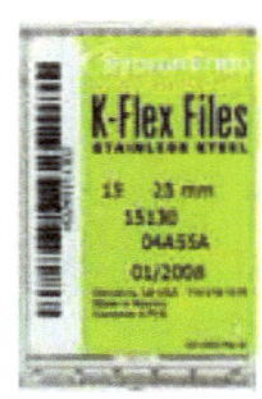

K-flex files

The cross-section of the k-flex is rhomboid or diamond-shaped. This new cross-section presented significant changes in the flexibility and cutting characteristics.

2) FlexO File

These instruments have a unique, silicone handle. The large, ergonomic handle provides comfort and excellent tactile feedback. It has x-ray-visible calibration rings (25 & 31mm) that help improve accuracy and diagnosis, and a stainless-steel triangular core file and safe-ended batt tip.

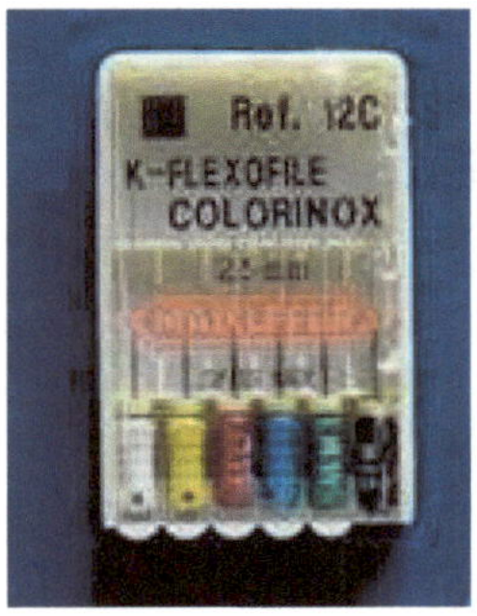

Flex-O file

Outstanding flexibility, cutting efficiency and unique non-slip handles make this the flexible file of choice for curved and narrow canals.

Use of Modified Tips

Flex-R files

Roane and Sabala[31] in 1988 confirmed that the modified non-end cutting tips exert less perforation and more inner curvature preparations. Powell and Simon put forward that metallic memory of the files returns to a straight position and increases the tendency for perforations. This action takes place in the outer curvature of the canal. They pointed out that when the tip angle is modified by reducing the tip angle, the file is centred within the canal and cuts all the walls more evenly.

Some of the modified tips commercially available:

1) Control safe file

2) Anti-ledging tip file

3) Safety hedstroem file.

H - File modification

Levy modified the Hedstroem file to function better with the automated canal finder system and named it as A file[1]. It is also supplied as a hand file. The unique features of this A file are its steep depth of flute and 40-degree helical angle of the cutting blade, which cuts more efficiently than the standard 60-degree or 70-degree helical angle.

Levy also pointed out that the steep blades on the inner curvature of the inner wall collapse and lose much of their cutting efficiency. The blades on the external wall open up and more aggressively attack the dentin. This is particularly effective in preparing the curved mesial canals of the lower molars, where the inner wall is more often stripped.

The non-cutting tip of this instrument also ensures that the point will follow the canal lumen and will not catch in the convex outer wall, resulting in ledging or perforations.

U Files

It is a new endodontic classification of instruments. It does not have any ISO, ANSI or ADA specifications. U file is developed by Heath and marketed as canal master U files, NiTi mac and ultra flex files.

The cross-section of these files is triangular, but with two 90-degree cutting edges at each point of the triangular blade. Health pointed out that the new U shape adapts well to the curved canal, it aggressively cuts the external convex wall while avoiding the more dangerous internal concave wall, where perforations or stripping occur.

The non-cutting tip of the U file ensures that the file remains in the lumen of the canal and avoids perforations at the apical segment.

Nickel titanium files:

More flexible file systems were also developed by making changes in the metal form. Instead of carbon steel or stainless steel, nickel-titanium was introduced for endodontic use, called NiTi files. These instruments have the ability to return to the original shape even if bent severely and held in this position for a long time. Because they have little resistance to pressure, the NiTi files cause little change in canal shape and the chance of producing ledges and perforation is minimised.

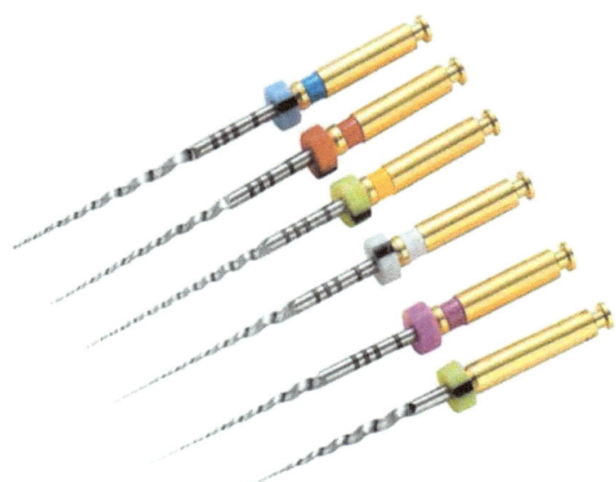

Protaper NiTi files

<u>Canal preparation techniques:</u>

Though several techniques have been advocated for biomechanical preparation, debate remains as to which technique is better for instrumentation of complex canals in order to prevent instrumentation errors.

Roane and Sabala introduced balanced force concept[31] of root canal preparation with the introduction of flex -R- files. It involves placement, cutting and removal using only rotary motions. Insertion is done with a half-turn clockwise rotation, and it should not exceed 180 degrees and counter-clockwise rotation with apical pressure is 120 degrees or greater. In this way, the instrument is advanced towards the apex. Studies have found that this technique is very effective for the treatment of curved canals.

Ultrasonic canal preparation

In 1957, Richman reported the use of barbed broaches connected to the ultrasonic system. In 1980, Martin, Cunningham and their group in Washington reported studies on many aspects of ultrasonic treatments. They coined the term endosonics.

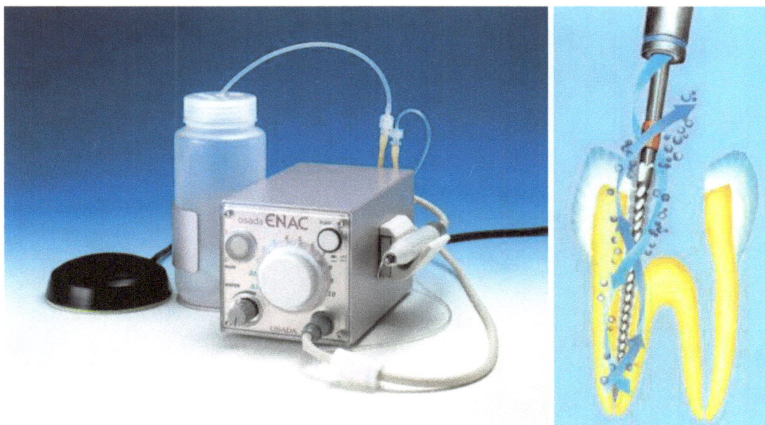

ENAC Ultrasonic Unit

Ultrasonics was initially described as implosion and cavitation. Cavitation occurs when the ultrasonic instruments produce vibrations in liquid to produce alternating compressions and rarefactions of pressure. A negative pressure develops with the exposed cells of the intracanal materials, which causes implosion or inward explosion.

But later, Ahmed and her group from Guys ' Hospital reported another mechanism. They reported that the power setting used to energise the ultrasonic unit is too low to produce cavitation, and the width of the canal is too small to allow for this condition. They stated that the principle used is acoustic streaming, a process by which the vibrating file generates a stream of liquid to produce eddies and flows of oscillations.

The energy from the ultrasonic device is from instruments vibrating at the level of 20 to 30 kHz by either electromagnetic or piezoelectric power sources. The frequently used ultrasonic electromagnetic unit is Cavi endo; the most used piezoelectric unit is ENAC.

Schultz et al suggested that when used alone in the canal with a curvature of 30 degrees or greater, severe zipping occurred. They suggested the use of ultrasonics in combination with hand instruments at the apex.

SEPARATED INSTRUMENTS AND FOREIGN OBJECTS

A separated root canal instrument is seldom, if ever, the sole cause of failure.

Since instruments are made of stainless steel or nickel-titanium alloy, it would be extremely rare for these materials to cause periradicular inflammation. Usually, the instrument is advanced into the canal until it binds, and efforts to remove it lead to breakage, leaving a segment of it in the canal; a stressed instrument may also cause the same problem.

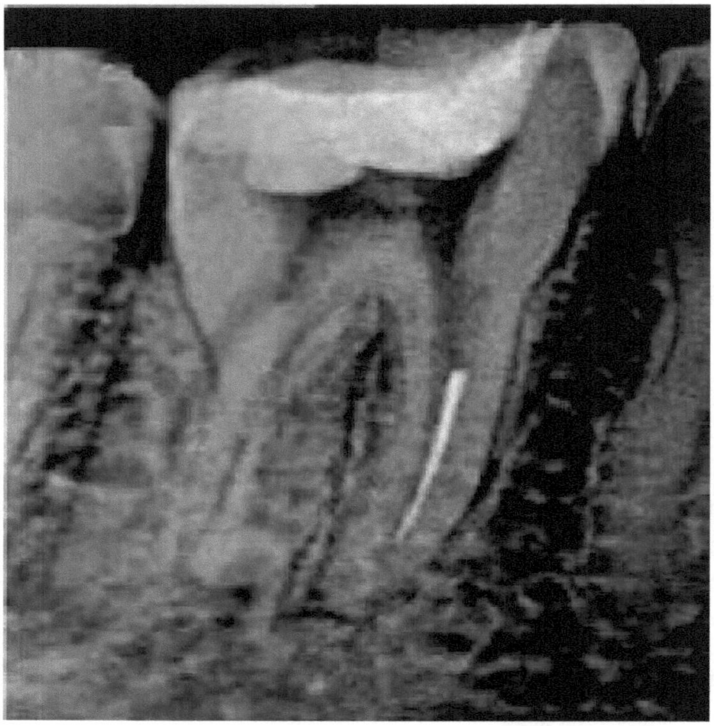

Separated instrument

Glass beads from sterilisers, burs, Gates-Glidden drills, amalgam, lentulo spiral, files and reamers, and tips of dental instruments have all found their way into canals, complicating treatment. Chenail and Teplitsky reviewed intra- and patient-placed foreign objects and listed, in addition to the above, nails, pencil lead, tooth picks, tomato seeds, hat pins, needles, pins, and other metal objects and advocated use of orthograde ultrasonics for removal.

The real problem is that the separated instrument blocks proper cleaning, shaping, and canal obturation. When these instruments can be removed, successful retreatment invariably ensues. Although it is possible to remove many of these instrument fragments, the majority will not be removable because of canal curvature or total blockage of the lumen, which prevents bypassing of the segment. Occasionally, it may be possible to bypass a fractured instrument segment and yet not be able to remove it. In these cases, the canal is cleaned, shaped and obturated, incorporating the fractured segment into the filling. Alternative treatment planning generally includes periradicular surgery or root or tooth resection.

Most commonly, files and reamers are involved in these types of procedural errors. Usually, the instrument is advanced into the canal until it binds, and efforts to remove it then lead to breakage, leaving a segment of it in the canal. Other common errors leading to this error are using a "stressed" instrument, placing exaggerated bends on instruments to negotiate curved canals, and forcing a file down a canal before the canal has been prepared sufficiently with the previous, smaller file and then using it in a reaming motion. The result is fracturing of the instrument.

Rotary instruments, such as Gates-Glidden drills, if stressed, will break close to the shank, leaving a piece that can be grasped and easily retrieved. The Stieglitz forceps are especially useful for this. If the break occurs closer to the bur head, retrieval is much more difficult.

The optimal correction of instrument fracture or the presence of other foreign objects in a canal is to remove the obstruction. As a general rule, efforts to remove instrument fragments should be made as the initial approach to corrective treatment. Ultrasonic fine instruments have proven most effective in loosening and flushing out broken fragments.

Use of ultrasonic devices is advocated in two different case reports wherein a tunnel is created around the separated instrument and a sleeve is positioned in the canal and around the separated instrument. In one study, cyanoacrylate is used to bind and remove the instrument, and in the other, an H-file is wedged in the sleeve until the instrument is locked between the flutes of the file and the wall of the sleeve. The efficacy of these techniques can be judged only based on the few case reports presented and may be attempted with no predictably favourable result. Recently, Hulsmann reported on the successful use of the canal finder system in combination with ultrasonic devices in bypassing and removing fractured instruments.

Actually, the prognosis may not be reduced at all. The presence of a separated instrument in the canal itself does not predispose the case to post-treatment disease. Rather, it is the presence of necrotic, infected pulp tissue that remains in the apical space that determines the prognosis.

The potential to remove a separated instrument depends on many factors, as the location of the separated instrument is of critical importance. If the instrument extends into the straight canal, retrieval is likely. If it has separated deep inside the canal and the entire broken segment is apical to the canal curvature, then orthograde removal will not be possible. If there is persistent disease and the file cannot be bypassed safely, either apical surgery or extraction will be necessary.

The type of material the separated instrument is made of will affect the chances of removal. NiTi files tend to shatter when ultrasonic energy is applied to them, hindering removal, whereas stainless steel instruments are more robust and more easily removed with ultrasonics.

Techniques for removal of separated instruments[32]

Many different techniques and instruments are available, all of which are very important for separated instrument removal. None, however, is more important than the operating microscope. This instrument not only increases visibility by the use of magnification and light but also increases the efficiency and safety of almost all the techniques discussed, and it is advisable not to attempt any of these techniques without the use of this valuable tool.

If the file is clinically visible in the coronal access and can be grasped with an instrument, such as a hemostat or Steiglitz pliers, these should be used to obtain a firm hold of the file and extract it through the access cavity preparation. However, establishing a firm purchase can be difficult without removing excess tooth structure. Once a purchase is made on the file has been achieved, it is best to pull it from the canal with a slight counterclockwise action. This action will unscrew the flutes that are engaged in the dentin as the file is being removed. This is the easiest way of removing a separated file; unfortunately, many files separate at a point where these forceps cannot be used.

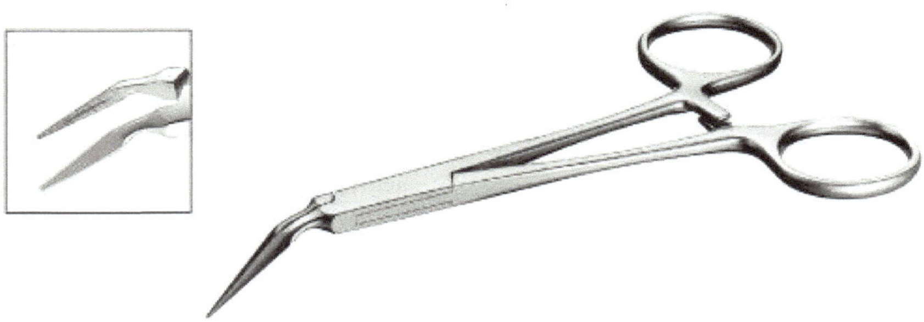

Steiglitz pliers

Frequently, a file will separate at a point deeper in the canal, where visibility is difficult. In order to remove separated root canal instruments predictably, the clinician must create straight-line coronal-radicular access. Either removing the crown or creating a large access cavity preparation establishes adequate coronal access to allow the use of the appropriate instruments. This can be created by using Gates-Glidden drills. This process will create a circumferential staging platform to facilitate ultrasonic use.

Ultrasonic technique

Ultrasonic instruments are very effective in the removal of canal obstructions [33, 34]. The ultrasonic tip is placed on the staging platform between the exposed end of the file and the canal wall and is vibrated. This technique will help in removing instruments that have a clockwise cutting action.

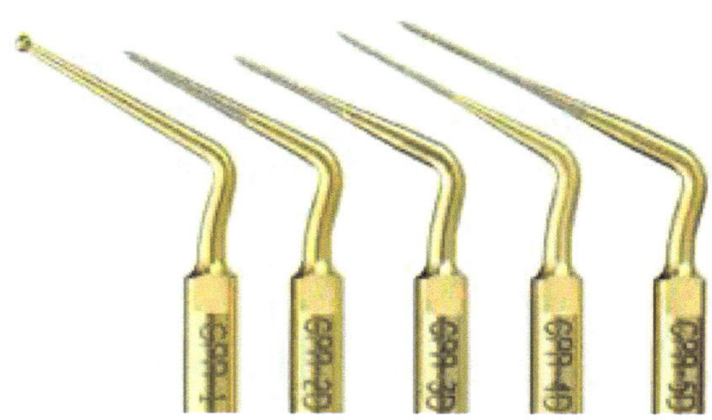

CPR ultrasonic tips

If the file had a counterclockwise cutting action, then a clockwise rotation is needed. The energy applied will aid in loosening the file, and occasionally the file will appear to jump out of the canal.

So it is good to cover the adjacent canals with cotton. Many different sizes and angles of tips are available. But in general, the deeper in the canal the obstruction is, the longer and thinner an ultrasonic tip must be. Occasionally, if the separated instrument can be bypassed, ultrasonic files can loosen it.

NiTi instruments often break up into fragments when subject to the energy supplied by an ultrasonic instrument. There is a chance of pushing the separated file further into the canal or beyond the apical foramen, which may increase the risk of this technique.

If the direct application of ultrasonic energy does not loosen the separated instrument sufficiently to remove it, the fragment must be grabbed and retrieved.

Simple Microtube Technique

This uses a short piece of stainless steel tubing that is pushed over the exposed end of the object. A small Hedstroem file is then pushed between the tube and the end of the object using a clockwise turning motion that produces a good mechanical lock among the separated instrument, the tube, and the H file. The three connected objects can then be removed by pulling them in a coronal direction.

The Endo Extractor Kit[35]

This includes a cyanoacrylate adhesive that is used to bond a hollow tube to the exposed end of the file for removal. This kit also includes four sizes of trephine burs and extractors. The most important factor in using this kit is the snugness of fit between the extractor tube and the obstruction. It has been shown that even with only 1mm of overlap between the extractor tube and the obstruction, if there is a snug fit, the bond created with the cyanoacrylate may be strong enough to remove many obstructions. However, the recommended amount of overlap is 2 mm. The time needed for the adhesive to set to ensure adequate bond strength for removal is 5 minutes for a snug fit and 10 minutes for a loose fit.

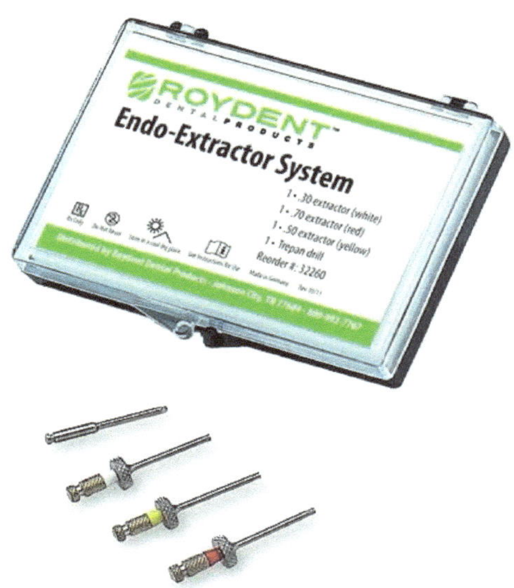

Endoextractor kit

Disadvantages:

1. The trephine burs are much larger than the ISO equivalents, so the manufacturer has added a separate, smaller trephine bur, which is sold separately from the kit.

2. The burs cut aggressively when new but dull rather quickly. This may result in perforation or even separation of the obstruction.

3. Once the separated instrument has been removed, the extractors may be reused, either by using the debonding agent that is included in the kit to remove the embedded instrument from the extractor tube or by simply cutting the extraction device with a bur beyond the extent that the separated instrument has penetrated.

The Masserann Technique

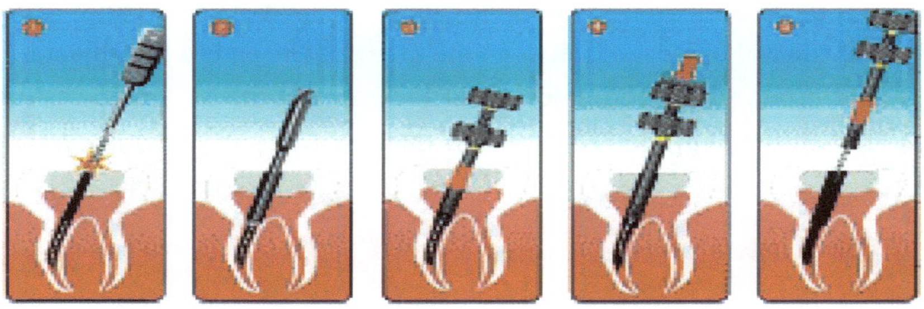

This technique is similar to the Endo Extractor in that it uses trephine burs and a specific extraction device. This kit comes with a very convenient gauge that aids in predicting the size of the bur and the extractor to be used, and it contains many different sizes of trephine burs. These burs cut in a counterclockwise direction, which provides an unscrewing force on separated files. The extraction mandrels have an internal stylus that wedges the file against the internal wall of the mandrel, allowing the obstruction to be removed. Although effective, this technique may require the removal of an excessive amount of radicular dentin, leading to root weakening and the risk of perforation. This instrument should be used with caution.

The Extractor system from Roydent

This system comes with only one bur and three extraction devices. The bur is very conservative and removes a minimal amount of tooth structure, enabling access to obstructions. The extractor tubes are also quite small and therefore will only work for the removal of small obstructions. The extractor surrounds the obstruction with six prongs that can be tightened onto the object, enabling removal. This works in the same way that a drill chuck tightens onto a drill bit. The disadvantages of this kit are the lack of variety of instruments, the possibility of separating the obstruction with the bur, and the potential problem of breakage of the prongs in the extractor if they are subjected to bending rather than applying strict tensile force during removal.

Instrument removal system

This kit consists of two different sizes of extraction devices that are tubes with a 45-degree bevel on the end and a side cutout window. Each tube has a corresponding internal stylus or screw wedge. Before the use of this instrument, 2 to 3 mm of the obstruction is exposed by making a trough around it with an ultrasonic instrument. Once the file is exposed by making a trough, the appropriate size microtube is selected and slid into place over the obstruction. Once in place, the screw wedge is turned counterclockwise to engage and displace the head of the obstruction through the side window. The assembly is then removed. This instrument is very useful in the straight portion of the canal, but it is difficult to force large-diameter separated files through the cutout window, hampering their removal.

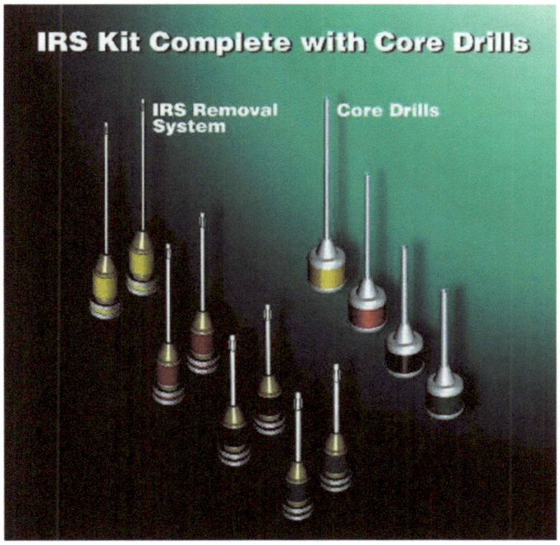

Instrument removal system

Separated Instrument Retrieval System (S.I.R)

This system is another microtube method of separated instrument retrieval. It uses extractor tubes bonded onto an obstruction, enabling removal. Once the obstruction is exposed using ultrasonics or the trephine burs, the bondable, dead soft tubes are bonded onto it. Once the adhesive is set, the obstruction is removed through the access cavity preparation. Included in this kit are the necessary bonding agent, a bottle of accelerator, five different sizes of tubes, assorted fulcrum props, and a hemostat. The accelerator causes the bonding agent to set almost instantaneously. The ability to bend these tubes allows for access in most areas of the mouth. A hemostat allows the clinician to establish a firm purchase on the tube, creating the ability to lever the bonded obstruction out of the canal. A vinyl autoclavable instrument prop provides protection for the next most anterior teeth, which is to be used as a fulcrum; however, if the clinician has access to grasp the extractor with the fingers to remove the extractor/obstruction unit, the hemostat may not be necessary.

Failing removal of the separated instrument, one of the following steps may be taken:

1. If the instrument fragment is totally within the root canal system, one may attempt to bypass it with a small file or reamer. Often, the instruments that break do so along the walls of the canal, being stuck between irregularities of secondary dentin or calcifications. Broken instruments can often be bypassed if the canals are oval or irregular in shape. Bypassing is made easier with a lubricant. If successful, the canal preparation can be completed and the canal filled regardless of whether the instrument segment is removed during the process of canal preparation. The instrument

segment thus becomes part of the filling material. The effort to bypass a broken instrument has its own risk: possible perforation of the canal.

2. If the fragment cannot be bypassed, one can prepare and fill the canal to the level at which instrumentation can be accomplished. As long as the separated instrument fragment is not protruding through the apex, further treatment, such as apical surgery, may not be necessary. The instrument itself, if embedded in the dentin before fragmentation, may help to seal the canal. Studies by Crump and Natkin and by Fox et al. have shown that success following instrument separation is equal to that of teeth without such errors.

3. If the fragment extends past the apex and efforts to remove it nonsurgically are unsuccessful, the corrective treatment will probably include apical surgery. The first step, though, will be to completely clean, shape and fill the canal. Following that, apical surgery would include removal of the part of the instrument fragment that extends beyond the apex and retrofilling if indicated.

Prognosis for a tooth with a separated instrument may not change very much if the instrument can be bypassed. If surgical correction is needed, the prognosis may be reduced depending on the outcome of the corrective treatment.

Prevention of separation errors can be partially accomplished by careful handling of instruments. Some instruments, however, will break even with cautious handling and utmost care.

The following is a list of guidelines for when to discard and replace instruments.

1. Flaws, such as shiny areas or unwinding, are detected on the flutes.

2. Excessive use has caused instrument bending or crimping, which is common with smaller-sized instruments. A major concern with nickel-titanium instruments is that they tend to fracture without warning; as a result, constant monitoring of usage is critical.

3. Excessive bending or precurving has been necessary.

4. Accidental bending occurs during file usage.

5. The file kinks instead of curving.

6. Corrosion is noted on the instrument.

7. Compacting instruments have defective tips or have been excessively heated. A separated instrument does not necessarily mean surgery or loss of the tooth.

8. Small instruments, such as Nos. 08, 10, 15, and 20 should be examined carefully during use to check for signs of stress.

9. Instruments No. 08 and 10 should be used only once. These smaller instruments should not be forced or wedged into a canal; rather, they should be teased gently into place.

According to Ingle[1], two important points will aid in the prevention of separation.

1. Sequential instrumentation, using the "quarter-turn" technique and increasing file size only after the current working file fits loosely into the canal without binding.
2. The gradual increase in file sizes, even including the currently available half-sizes, and avoiding the rush to finish, will go a long way toward preventing errors.

CANAL BLOCKADE

When a canal suddenly does not permit a working file to be advanced to the apical stop, a situation sometimes referred to as a blockout has occurred. Buchanan states that blockage occurs when files compact apical debris into a hardened mass. He further noted that fibrous blockage occurs when vital pulp tissue is compacted and solidified against the apical constriction.

Recognition occurs when the confirmed working length is no longer attained. Evaluation radiographically will demonstrate that the file is not near the apical terminus.

Correction is accomplished by recapitulation. Starting with the smallest file, the quarter-turn technique is used; using a chelating agent can be helpful. If the blockout occurs at a curve or bend of the root, gently precurving the instruments to redirect it is also effective. Caution must be employed in attempting to recover from a blockout occurring at a curve or bend. An all too common and unfortunate result is the creation of a ledge and/or lateral perforation. Precurving instruments during the redirection process and radiographic confirmation are essential.

Prognosis depends on the stage of instrumentation completed when the blockout occurs. If the canal has been adequately cleaned, it should have little or no effect. If, however, the blockout occurs before the canal is clean, the prognosis will be reduced. Teeth with vital pulps have a better prognosis than those with necrotic pulps.

Prevention consists of recapitulation during canal preparation to remove dentin debris. The use of water-soluble lubricants such as File Eze or K-Y Jelly is also a preventive measure.

OBTURATION-RELATED ERRORS

OVER OR UNDEREXTENDED ROOT CANAL FILLINGS

Although controversy still may exist regarding apical termination of the root canal filling, there is general agreement that the ideal location is at or near the dentino-cemental junction. Many studies have supported the apical termination of the filling material just short of the radiographic apex.

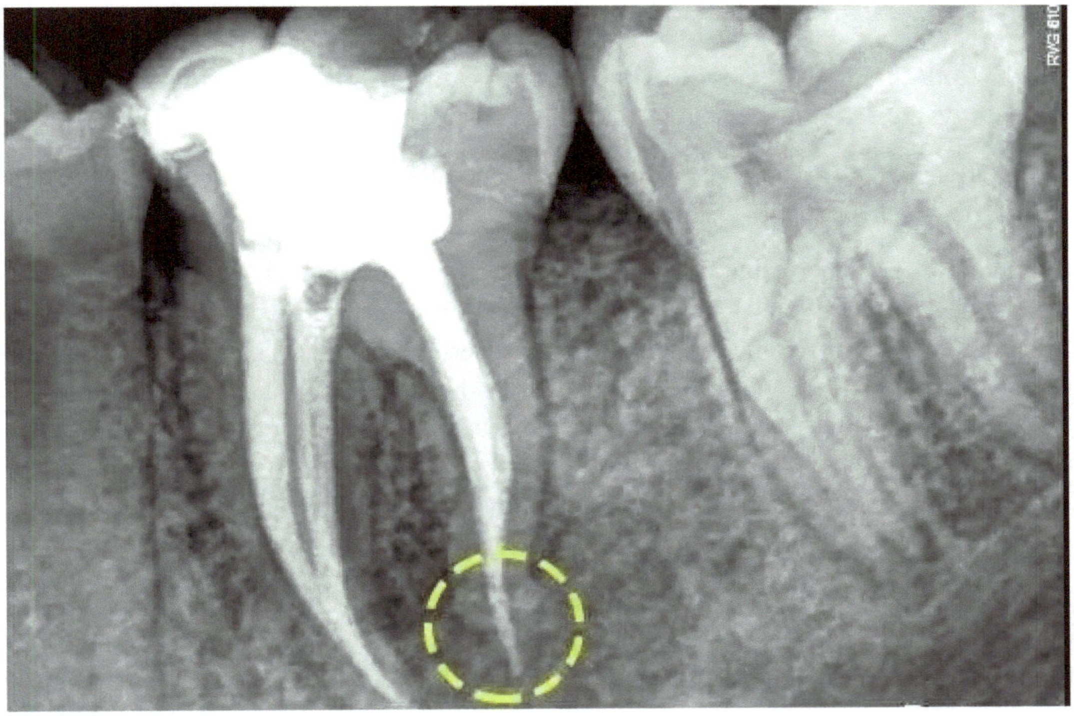

Over extension

Root canal filling material is sometimes inadvertently extruded beyond the apical limit of the root canal system, ending up in the periradicular bone, sinus, or mandibular canal, or even protruding through the cortical plate. Gross overextensions can lead to symptoms and treatment failure. A frequent cause of this error is loss of apical constriction against which gutta-percha is compacted. Treatment failure may be less from irritation of the filling material and more from leakage around a poorly compacted filling. Roane and associates have attempted to minimise apical canal transportation, a frequent cause of overextrusion of root canal filling, by use of the "balance forced" approach[31, 36]. The results have been promising.

Underextension of root canal filling material may be caused by failure to fit the master gutta-percha point accurately. It can also result from a poorly prepared canal, particularly in the apical part of the canal.

Extruded pastes can also lead to complications. Case reports citing materials such as N2, Hydron, AH26, Diaket, and even zinc oxide-eugenol-based sealers have been published. These articles have shown that, in addition to the effects of the material, the sequelae and untoward effects are location-related. The risk of this occurrence rises in the root canal, wherein the apical stop is inadequately prepared. Rowe stated that, in teeth with apices approximating the inferior alveolar canal, a frequent cause of damage is excess filling material which has passed through the apices and either caused pressure on the neurovascular bundle in the inferior dental canal or produced a neurotoxic effect on the nerve trunk. Overextension of materials into the alveolar cancellous bone near other teeth that are not close to a sensory nerve can also be expected to produce mild to moderate or severe discomfort until the initial inflammatory response subsides.

Recognition of an inaccurately placed root canal filling usually takes place when a post-treatment radiograph is examined.

Correction of an under-extended filling is accomplished by re-treatment: removal of the old filling followed by proper preparation and obturation of the canal. Correction of an over-extended filling is more difficult. An attempt to remove the over-extension is sometimes successful if the entire point can be removed with one tug. Many times, however, the point will break off, leaving a fragment loose in the periradicular tissue. Attempts at removing a laterally condensed overextension, by using chloroform and a Hedstroem file, will usually produce the same results as trying to retrieve an overextended thermoplastic filling material; it may be pushed further into the periradicular tissue. If the overextended filling cannot be removed through the canal, it will be necessary to remove the excess surgically if symptoms or radicular lesions develop or increase in size.

Root canal filling materials such as gutta-percha and many sealers are generally well tolerated by the surrounding tissues, and overextended fillings do not automatically require surgical removal if asymptomatic and not associated with lesions. If symptoms persist from a tooth with an overextended gutta-percha filling, surgical removal of the excess material is usually a relatively minor procedure. If the root canal has been adequately cleaned and filled, a retrofilling is not necessary.

In re-treatments, the material being removed and the method of removal both affect the potential for overextension and extent of damage to the surrounding tissues. Spangberg studied the effect of various root canal filling materials on HeLa cells and found that amalgam, gutta-percha, and zinc phosphate had the least toxic effect, followed by calcium hydroxide paste, AH26 and Tubliseal. Chloropercha, Diaket, and N2 had the strongest toxicity.

The effects of over- or underextensions on prognosis vary. Care should be taken in obtaining good apical seals. Consequently, if the overextended filling provides an adequate seal, treatment may still be successful. In cases of under-extended fillings, the prognosis depends on the presence or absence of a periradicular lesion and the content of the root canal segment that remains unfilled.

If a lesion is present or the apical canals have necrotic or infected material in them, the prognosis diminishes considerably without re-treatment.

Attention to detail is the best form of prevention. Accurate working lengths and care to maintain them will help prevent over-extensions. Modifying the obturation technique may also be preventive. In younger patients with wider root canal systems or in teeth with apical resorption, the apical stop may not be adequate to prevent gutta-percha from being extruded. Techniques that create apical barriers with calcium hydroxide, dentin chips, or MTA may be useful in these cases.

Incorporation of two simple steps into one's root canal treatment technique can significantly decrease the chance of aberrant fillings: first, confirmation and adherence to canal working length throughout the instrumentation procedure, and second, taking a radiograph during the initial phases of the obturation to allow for corrective action.

NEUROLOGICAL COMPLICATIONS OF ENDODONTIC TREATMENT

Neurological complications are a recognised complication of endodontic treatment, particularly when there is injury to the inferior alveolar nerve, mental nerve, or, less commonly, the lingual nerve.

Aspect	Details
Primary causes	Overextension of root canal filling materials• Over-instrumentation beyond the apical foramen
Mechanism	Over-instrumentation may perforate the mandibular canal, allowing extrusion of sealers, irrigants, intracanal medicaments, and microorganisms into the canal, leading to nerve injury.
Clinical manifestations	Anaesthesia – Complete loss of sensation Paraesthesia – Abnormal sensation (tingling, "pins and needles") Hypoesthesia – Reduced sensation Hyperesthesia – Increased sensitivity Dysesthesia – Painful or unpleasant abnormal sensation
Neurotoxic materials	Eugenol, Paraformaldehyde (N2, Endomethasone), AH-26, Hydron, Diaket, Iodoform, Calasept, Endoseal, and Chloro-percha can cause serious neurotoxic effects if extruded into the mandibular canal.
Management – Minor overextension	Usually requires periodic observation and follow-up, as most cases resolve without intervention.
Management – Symptomatic nerve injury	Conservative management with observation is the initial approach. Systemic prednisone may be prescribed to reduce inflammation, minimise fibrosis, and shorten recovery (Gatot & Tovi).
Surgical management	Decompression surgery is indicated in persistent or severe nerve compression and may result in complete resolution of anaesthesia or paraesthesia.
Importance of early intervention	Prolonged contact of root canal sealer with the nerve can cause ischemia → epineural oedema → connective tissue proliferation → epineural fibrosis, reducing the chance of recovery.

Aspect	Details
Prognosis	Russell et al. reported complete recovery from anaesthesia when decompression surgery was performed within 3 days of injury.

VERTICAL ROOT FRACTURES

Vertical root fractures can occur during different phases of treatment[28] instrumentation, obturation, and post placement. In both lateral and vertical compaction techniques, the risk of fracture is high if too much force is exerted during compaction. Similarly, during placement, if the post is forced apically during seating or cementation, the risk of fracture is high, particularly if the post is tapered.

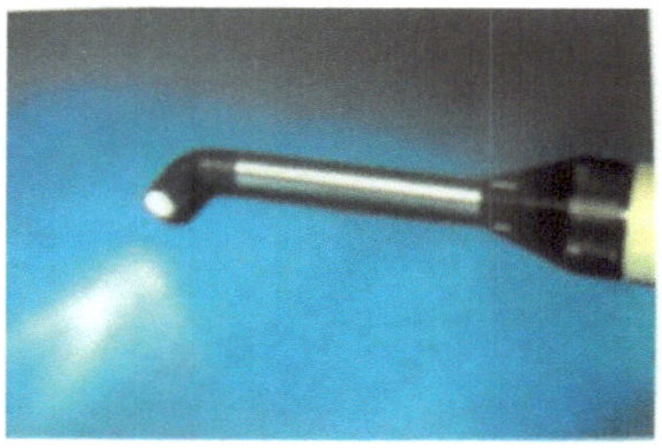

Fibreoptic light to detect vertical fracture

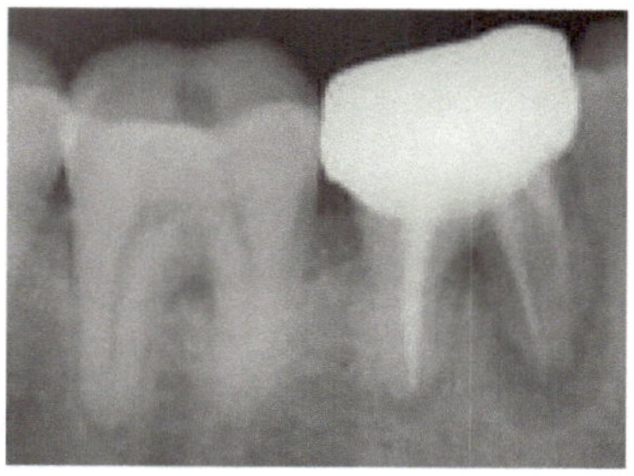

Vertical fracture in the lower second molar

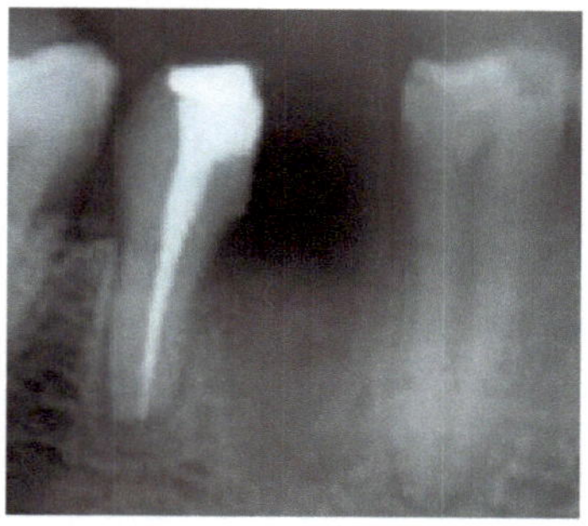

After hemisection

The sudden crunching sound similar to that referred to as crepitus in the diseased temporomandibular joint, accompanied by pain reaction on the part of the patient, is a clear indicator that the root has fractured. Suggestive "teardrop" radiolucency may appear in the radiographs of long-standing vertical root fracture and may be associated with only minor symptoms of soreness in the tooth. To confirm the diagnosis of a vertical fracture, exploratory surgery is a good way to visualise the fracture, but a deep periodontal pocket of recent origin in a tooth with a long-present root canal filling is most suggestive of a vertical root fracture.

Unfortunately, in most cases of vertical fracture, extraction is the only treatment available at this time. Glass ionomer cement repairs for furcal perforations have been reported by Alhadainy and Himel. The bonding ability of glass ionomer cement and dentin bonded resins[39,40] has led other investigators to use it in attempts to repair vertical root fractures. A 1-year success was reported in a single case[41].

Sugaya T [40] (2001) clinically evaluated the periodontal healing of root fracture treatment using adhesive resin cement. The results suggested that treatment of vertical root fractures with 4-META/MMA-TBB resin has good prognostic potential.

Vertical root fracture treated by bonding fragments and rotational replantation has been reported by Kawai K et al. ([42] (2002). These case reports describe a new treatment method for complete vertical root fractures. This method is composed of two steps. First, the fractured tooth is intentionally extracted atraumatically, and then the separated fragments are bonded with adhesive resin cement. The restored tooth is replanted by rotating approximately 180 degrees into the original socket and fixing it with an orthodontic wire. For both cases reported here, bone regeneration was observed at the 3-year follow-up. Since this modality adopts the respective advantages of both intentional replantation and adhesive treatment, it might be the treatment of choice in cases of vertical root fracture.

Young Bui (2004) has reported a case report using MTA to treat a vertical fracture tooth.

Hayashi M[39] (2004) evaluated the long-term prognosis of the intentional replantation of 26 vertically fractured roots after reconstruction with 4 - META / MMA - TBB dentin-bonded resin. Longitudinal fractures extending more than 2/3 from the cervical portion toward the apex showed significantly shorter longevity compared with fractures within the 2/3 area. Intentional replantation of vertically fractured roots reconstructed with dentin-bonded resin may be considered for incisors as an alternative to extraction, although the long-term success is not optimal.

To date, no consistently successful techniques have been reported to correct this problem.

Because this error produces irreversible damage to the tooth, it is most important to recognise the causes and adjust the techniques that might cause them.

Prevention involves the avoidance of overpreparing canals and the use of a passive and less forceful obturation technique and seating of posts. In his study, Helfer et al concluded that endodontically treated teeth are more brittle. Tidmarsh[43] states that the change in architecture of an endodontically treated tooth requires a restoration that will protect the tooth from fracture during function. Hence, full cuspal coverage is recommended.

OTHER ERRORS

POST SPACE PERFORATION

A well-done root canal procedure can be destroyed in a few seconds by a misdirected post space preparation. Unfortunately, perforations are the common cause of failure when endodontically treated teeth are restored. These failures are mainly due to improper restorative concepts and poor clinical judgment.

The post should be long enough to satisfy clinical requirements without affecting the root integrity.

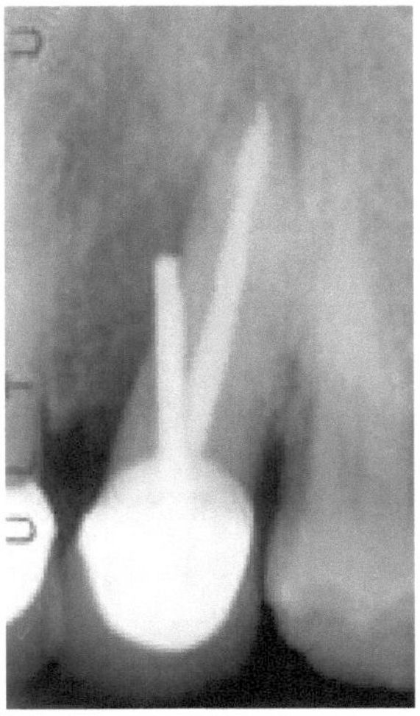

Post perforation in an anterior tooth

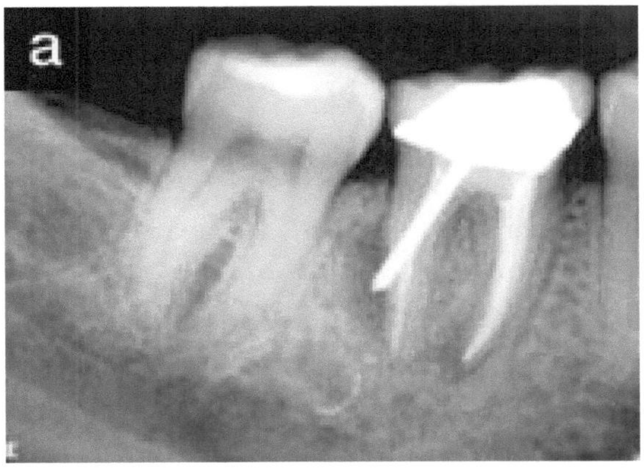

Post-perforation in the distal canal

The standard parameters used for the post space in the tooth with a normal periodontal support are.

1) Two third the length of the canal.
2) An amount equal to the coronal length of the tooth.
3) One-half the bone support length of the root.

Increasing the post space beyond 50% of the bone-encased root will increase the risk of perforations. The root should have more than 1mm of the remaining root structure circumferentially around the post to prevent perforations. The greater the curvature of the root and the more coronally located the curvature, the shorter the post should be placed to prevent perforations.

Maxillary first premolars have deep mesial concavities and a slender root with thin dentin. Maxillary first molars have deep concavities on the furcal surface of 94% of the mesiobuccal roots, 3% of the distobuccal roots and 17% of the palatal root. Mandibular first molars have concavities on the furcal surface; 100% of the mesial root and 99% of the distal root.

Despite the recommendation of 1mm of the remaining dentin in the post preparation procedures, the dentin thickness in the furcation of mandibular molars has been reported to be less than 1mm in 82% of endodontically treated cases.

Post space preparations should not enlarge the root canal at the expense of the dentin. GG drills of size more than no. 3 should not be used in the distal root of mandibular molars. Large post space does not increase retention, but it increases the chances of root perforations.

Maxillary premolars and mesial root of mandibular molars, which have an elliptical or ribbon shape, cannot be reshaped to accommodate a round post. In such cases, two small-diameter fibre posts can be adhesively cemented into the canal to give additional retention without affecting the integrity of the roots.

Use of parallel posts, especially in maxillary first premolar, mandibular central and lateral incisors, may perforate the lateral surface of the tooth. Consideration should be given to using a tapered post or a parallel post of a smaller size.

When the outline of the canal is oval, it is difficult to prepare a circular post channel to receive a parallel post; in that case, a custom-made post is preferred.

When a multirooted tooth has been endodontically treated, it is difficult to decide which root has to be considered for post placement. Mesial root of mandibular molars and buccal roots of maxillary molars are often curved, and they frequently present a problem in preparing the post space because of inadequate length and width. Perforations may result when these roots are chosen for post placement; therefore, the distal roots of mandibular molars and the palatal root of maxillary molars are best suited for post placement.

End-cutting drills such as those used for the Para post system need careful attention to avoid lateral perforation; round burs and tapered fissure burs can also be dangerous if care is not exercised in watching the direction of the bur.

Recognition is similar to that of instrumentation-related lateral root perforations: sudden presence of blood in the canal during post preparation or radiographic evidence.

Correction consists of sealing the perforation, as for any other perforations. The use of a resin composite bonded to adjacent root dentin with a dentin bonding agent has been reported for both retro root-filling material and as a retro sealing in root perforations associated with improper post placement.

Prognosis is least affected if the perforation is totally within bone; if it is closer to the gingival sulcus, the risk of pocket formation is high, but, in any case, the tooth must be considered weakened.

Prevention is associated with a good knowledge of root canal anatomy and planning the post space preparation based on radiographic information regarding the location of the root and its direction in the alveolus. Preparing the space at the time the root canal is obturated reduces the risk of perforation. It is safer to do so with a hot instrument or a file than with a round bur or an end-cutting bur. Gates-Glidden and Peeso drills are not likely to be at risk in causing perforation; however, they can lead to excessive removal of tooth structure and therefore can potentially lead to "stripping" or root fracture.

IRRIGANT-RELATED ERRORS

Various irrigants have been used in the chemomechanical preparation of the root canal system. Saline, hydrogen peroxide, alcohol, and sodium hypochlorite are amongst those most commonly used. Any irrigant, regardless of toxicity, has the potential to cause problems if extruded into periradicular tissues. The fear of the toxicity of sodium hypochlorite as an irritant of periradicular tissue has tended to deter its use. In one study, however, no significant inflammatory difference was noted after 7 to 24 days when solutions of sodium hypochlorite ranging from 8.4 to 0.9% were implanted in polyethene tubes into the backs of guinea pigs.

On the other hand, forcibly injecting sodium hypochlorite, or any irrigating solution, through the canal into the surrounding tissue is another matter entirely[44]. The number of cases reported probably does not truly reflect the incidence of this occurrence. Becker et al. described the damaging effects of an accidental injection of sodium hypochlorite beyond the apex.

Bhat[45] reported the same effects with hydrogen peroxide. Injection of hydrogen peroxide causes tissue emphysema.

Hypochlorite complications

NaOCl is tissue cytotoxic[46]. When it comes into contact with tissue, it causes hemolysis and ulceration, inhibits neutrophil migration, and damages endothelial and fibroblast cells[47].

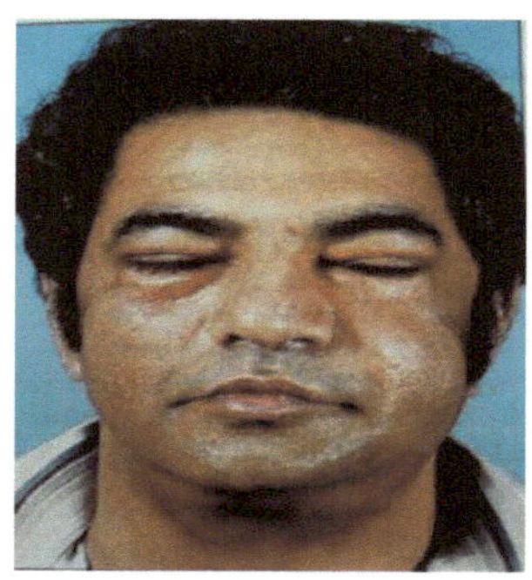

Hypochlorite accident-swelling

<u>Complications arising from hypochlorite extrusion beyond the root apex[48, 49, 50.]</u>

(1) Chemical burns and tissue necrosis

- Localised or extensive tissue necrosis
- A severe inflammatory reaction of the tissues develops that leads to rapid tissue swelling both intra- and extra-orally
- Swelling may be edematous, hemorrhagic or both
- Sudden onset of pain is a hallmark of tissue damage, and may occur immediately or be delayed for several minutes or hours
- Involvement of the maxillary sinus will lead to acute sinusitis

- Associated bleeding into the interstitial tissues results in bruising, ecchymosis or hematoma. [47]
- A necrotic ulceration of the mucosa adjacent to the tooth
- Treatment- urgent hospitalisation and administration of intravenous steroids and antibiotics

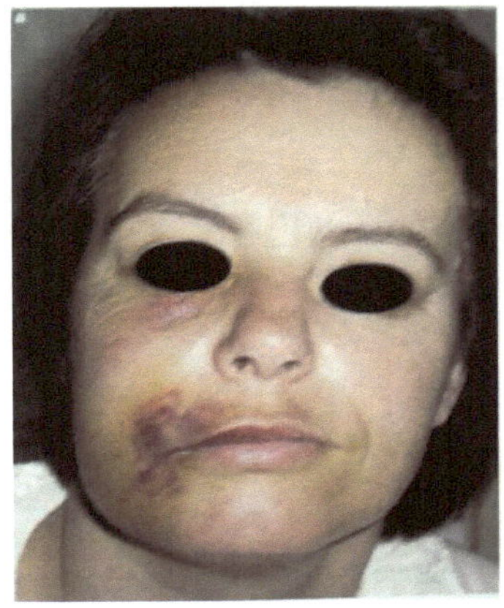

Hypochlorite accident-ecchymosis

(2) Neurological complications[51]

- Paraesthesia and anaesthesia affecting the mental, inferior dental and infraorbital branches of the trigeminal nerve following inadvertent extrusion of sodium hypochlorite beyond the root canals
- Normal sensation may take many months to completely resolve
- Facial nerve damage (Witton et al in, 2005), where the buccal branch of the facial nerve was affected

(3) Upper airway obstruction

- Leakage of the solution into the oral cavity and ingestion or inhalation by the patient may cause upper airway obstruction
- Reaction of toxic sodium hypochlorite entering the tissues
- A combination of periapical bone destruction (chronic infection) and increased pressure irrigation may lead to the entry of sodium hypochlorite into the adjacent soft tissues.
- It is also possible that intracanal bacteria may be carried into the tissues, thereby posing a potential infection risk.

Precautions

- A rubber dam should be used to isolate the tooth

- Side-vented needles should be used. (Monoject needles and Max-I probe) The use of hypodermic, end-exiting needles in root canal irrigation risks accidental inoculation into the soft tissues.

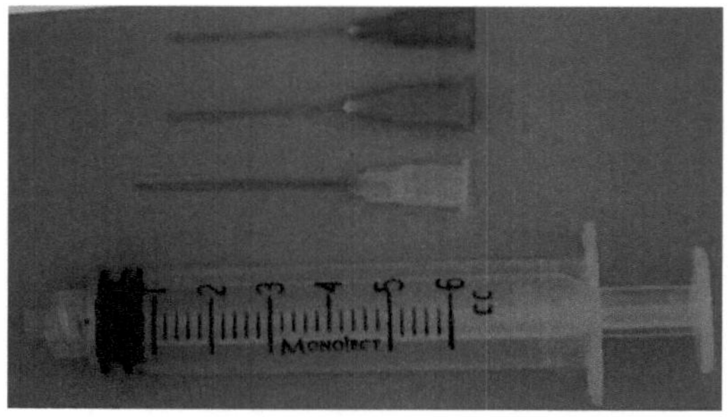

Monoject needle

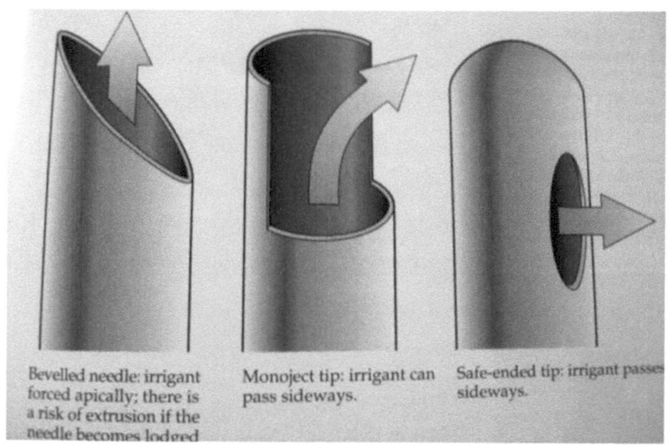

Only Luer-Lok syringes and needles should be used.

- Needle should not engage the sides of the canal
- Needle should not reach the apical extent of the prepared canal.
- Irrigant should be delivered with minimal pressure, and it is achieved by using the index finger rather than the thumb to depress the plunger.
- Particular care must be taken in immature teeth with open apices.

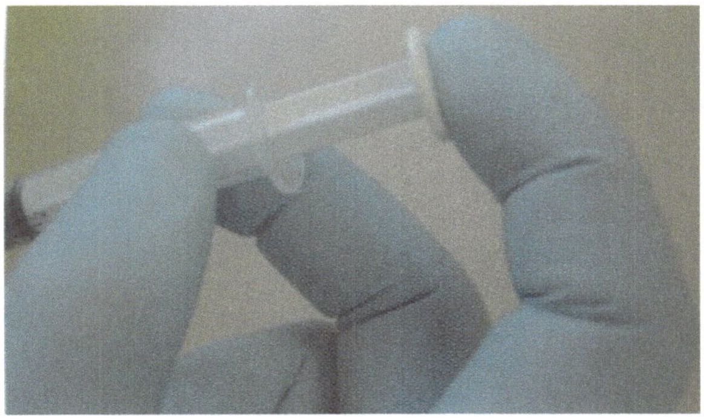

The index finger is used to depress the plunger.

Recognition

- Immediate severe pain for 2-6 minutes
- Ballooning or immediate oedema in adjacent soft tissue because of perfusion to the loose connective tissue
- Extension of oedema to a large site of the face, such as cheeks, periorbital region, or lips
- Ecchymosis on skin or mucosa as a result of profuse interstitial bleeding

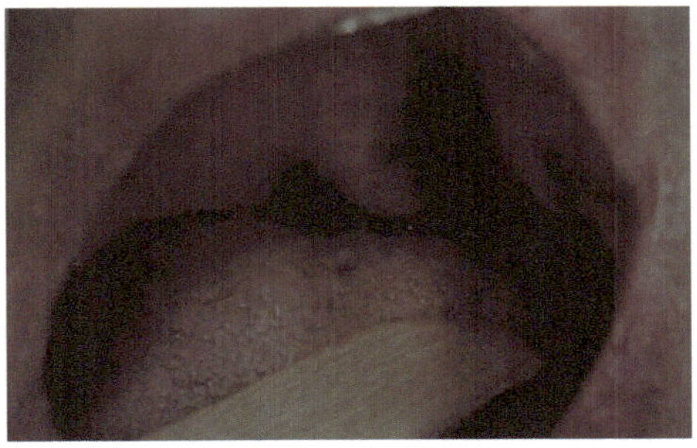

Ecchymosis extending into the soft palate

- Profuse intraoral bleeding directly from the root canal
- Chlorine taste or smell because of the injected NaOCl in the maxillary sinus
- Severe initial pain replaced with a constant discomfort or numbness, related to tissue destruction and distension
- Reversible or persistent anaesthesia.
- Possibility of secondary infection or spreading of the former infection.

Management

- Early recognition of the problem and informing the patient about the accident.
- Immediate irrigation of the canal with normal saline to dilute the NaOCl
- Allow bleeding response to continue as it helps to flush the irritant out of the tissues
- Patient should be reassured and provided with both verbal and written home care instructions
- Ice bag compresses should be advised for 24 hours, at 15-minute intervals, to minimise the swelling
- Warm moist compresses are advised after 24 hours
- Rinsing with normal saline is advised for 1 week to improve circulation to the affected area.
- Initial control of acute pain with anaesthetic nerve block
- Acetaminophen-based analgesics for 3-7 days. NSAID analgesics should be avoided to decrease the amount of bleeding into the soft tissues.
- Prophylactic antibiotic coverage for 7-10 days to prevent secondary infection or spreading of the present infection.
- Steroid therapy with methylprednisolone for 2-3 days to control the inflammatory reaction.
- The patient should be contacted daily to monitor recovery.
- In severe cases of respiratory distress, emergency medical services should be contacted.
- The patient should be reassured about the lengthy resolution of the inflammatory reaction.
- The patient should be monitored for pain control and secondary infection.

Allergy to sodium hypochlorite

Hypersensitivity to sodium hypochlorite may occur. A patient reported sensitivity to household bleach, and a forearm patch test confirmed it. Wisely, the dentist chose to use a substitute irrigant during endodontic therapy.

- First reported in 1940 by Sulzberger and subsequently by Cohen and Burns
- Non-allergic hypersensitivity - no immunological mechanism
- Skin scratch test useful (Kaufman and Keila)[52]
- Symptoms of allergy and possible anaphylaxis can occur
- Urgent referral to a hospital following first aid management is recommended.

TISSUE EMPHYSEMA

Subcutaneous or periradicular air emphysema is, fortunately, relatively uncommon. Tissue space emphysema has been defined as the passage and collection of gas in tissue reported as an untoward event subsequent to various dental procedures.

The common etiologic factor is compressed air being forced into the tissue spaces. Emphysema can occur when a blast of air is blown to dry the canal, or during surgery, air from a high-speed drill enters the tissue space. Injection of hydrogen peroxide into the periapex can also cause emphysema[45].

Recognition:

The usual sequence of events is rapid swelling, erythema, and crepitus. Hayduk et al. regard crepitus as a pathognomonic sign of tissue space emphysema. Although pain is not a major complaint, dysphagia and dyspnea have been reported. Unlike irrigant extrusion reactions, tissue space emphysema remains in the subcutaneous connective tissue and usually does not spread to the deep anatomic spaces.

Complications - pneumothorax, pneumopericardium, mediastinitis, life-threatening air embolism.

Treatment:

- Resolves after 2–3 days of supportive treatment, with complete resolution after 7–10 days.
- Observation for potential airway embarrassment, cardiovascular or infectious processes is often all that is required.
- Surgical decompression of extensive emphysema should not be routinely undertaken as it is not likely to be effective and may increase or spread the entrapped gas.
- The potential for infection is also a concern.
- Penicillin is an empirical first-choice antibiotic.
- Analgesics are prescribed as necessary.
- Reassurance
- Patients should be cautioned to return in the case of increased swelling or difficulty in breathing.

Prevention:

- Operative sites should be closely inspected and protected to reduce or prevent air from entering.
- Handpieces that exhaust air into the surgical field should not be used.
- Air-cooled instruments used in surgical orofacial procedures should vent air away from the immediate area or recirculate the air to reduce the risk of introducing it into tissues.
- The occurrence of sudden swelling during a dental procedure, marked by crepitus within the soft tissue, should raise suspicion of subcutaneous emphysema.

INSTRUMENT ASPIRATION AND INGESTION

Aspiration or ingestion of a foreign object is a complication that can occur during any dental procedure.

Endodontic instruments, used in the absence of a rubber dam, can easily be aspirated or swallowed if inadvertently dropped in the mouth. Case reports have been published with reamers or files located in either the food or air passages. The common denominator in all is failure to use a rubber dam. Mejia et al[53] reported a case of swallowing of a rubber dam clamp by the patient. The standard of care for endodontic therapy requires the use of a rubber dam. It is not an option not to use it. Practitioners performing endodontic therapy without the use of a rubber dam are placing themselves in unnecessary legal jeopardy. It should be considered that all intraoral procedures involve risks, and a rubber dam must be used.

Symptoms depend on where the object becomes impacted.

- Above the vocal cords→ acute respiratory distress.

Smaller objects do not produce upper airway obstruction.

- Laryngotracheal→ dyspnoea, cough, and stridor

Bronchial - cough, decreased air entry, dyspnoea, and wheezing.

- Hoarseness will accompany obstruction of the larynx or trachea with or without cyanosis, depending on whether the obstruction is partial or complete.

Secondary symptoms - pneumonia may develop.

- Foreign bodies that have been present for some time can cause abscess formation, pneumonia, atelectasis, or bronchiectasis, and their removal can be complicated by granulation or scar tissue.

The most readily visible sites for entrapment of a foreign body that has become displaced in the oropharynx are the supratonsillar recess, the epiglottic vallecula and the piriform recess.

If the foreign body cannot be found in these places, it should be assumed that it has either been swallowed or aspirated.

Aspiration or ingestion is an infrequent occurrence, and ingestion occurs more often.

Symptoms of oesophageal obstruction:

- inability to swallow, muscle incoordination, pain on swallowing, haematemesis, or vomiting.
- Symptoms of perforation vary between abdominal pain, fever, nausea, vomiting, abdominal distension and diagnosis can be difficult.

- traverse the intestinal tract → 2–12 days.
- Diet supplement→ large amount of cellulose, which theoretically will aid the passage of the object through the gut.
- Favoured by the small size of the instruments used by dentists and by the supine position of the patient.
- more frequent in selected groups, including prisoners, psychotics, alcoholics, mentally retarded hyperactive individuals and patients with excessive gag reflex

Diagnosis

- radiographs of the chest and abdomen.
- For radiolucent objects, ingestion of cotton wool pellets mixed with small amounts of barium sulphate suspension has been reported to form a radio-opaque bolus around the object, which allows it to be tracked through the gut radiographically.
- CT scanning and barium swallows
- Ultrasound
- If an object is swallowed, seek medical advice and refer for further investigation and possible early elective removal if there is a thought of an increased risk of perforation. It is also helpful to bring a sample file along so that the physician, who may be searching for an instrument in the alveolar tree, has a better idea of the size and shape of the instrument.

Precautions

- using a rubber dam

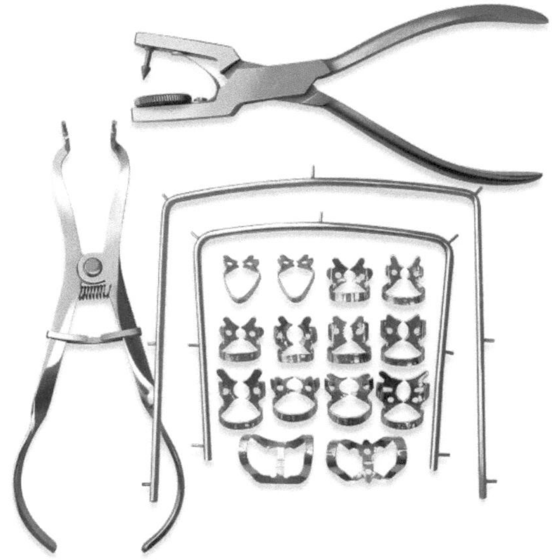

Rubber dam kit

- Tethering any small instrument with a ligature
- Placing a gauze screen to protect the oropharynx in sedated patients
- Innovative technique that involves adding a V-shaped loop to all castings to tether floss, which would help during the try-in phases for fixed prostheses (Ulusoy and Toksavul*).*
- Aspiration and ingestion are more likely to occur in this type of situation, and patients should not be reclined as far back in the chair as they are during other procedures.
- The impression material used should have a high viscosity, and the tray should be the correct size and fit.
- An upright position.
- The clinician should be able to visualise the back of the upper tray as it is seated in the mouth, so excess impression material is not allowed to extrude into the back of the mouth.

Management (Conscious patient):

Step	Management of Foreign Body Airway Obstruction (Conscious Patient)
1. Assess the patient	Confirm the patient is conscious and has signs of airway obstruction. Encourage coughing if the patient can cough effectively.
2. Retrieve visible foreign body	If the foreign body is clearly visible, remove it using hemostats or high-volume suction with a pharyngeal tip. Do not perform blind finger sweeps.
3. Allow the patient to cough	If the patient becomes agitated or attempts to sit up, allow them to do so—they may be trying to expel the foreign body by coughing.
4. Perform abdominal thrusts (Heimlich maneuver)	If the patient cannot cough effectively and the foreign body cannot be seen or removed, perform the Heimlich maneuver (abdominal thrusts).
5. Special situation	For pregnant patients (or when abdominal thrusts are contraindicated), perform 4 chest thrusts instead of abdominal thrusts.
6. Repeat as needed	Continue alternating thrusts until the foreign body is expelled or the patient becomes unconscious. If the patient becomes unconscious, immediately follow the unconscious patient airway obstruction protocol (Basic Life Support).
7. After successful removal	Administer 100% oxygen, monitor the patient's airway, breathing, and circulation, and arrange medical evaluation if indicated.

Management (Unconscious patient)

Step	Action
1	Check responsiveness: Shake the shoulder and shout, "Are you okay?"
2	Lay the patient flat: Do not keep the patient sitting, as this may reduce cerebral circulation.
3	Open the airway: Perform the head tilt-chin lift maneuver.
4	Check breathing: Look, listen, and feel for breath for a few seconds.
5	Attempt to ventilate: If breathing is absent, try to give rescue breaths.
6	If the airway is obstructed: Reposition the head and try again.
7	If obstruction persists: Turn the victim toward you and give firm back blows between the shoulder blades.
8	Abdominal thrusts: Perform abdominal thrusts if the airway remains blocked.
9	Reposition the head again: Open the airway and reassess.
10	Repeat the sequence: Continue the cycle if the obstruction is not relieved.

Whenever a foreign body cannot be located, the operator should assume it has been swallowed until proven otherwise.[42]

Procedures for Questionable Swallowing or Aspiration of Foreign Body

1. Do not panic and do not leave the patient unattended.

2. Inform the instructor and mobilize portable emergency unit. Alert the Oral Surgery Emergency Team.

3. The patient may not be aware of swallowing or aspirating a foreign body. If the patient becomes agitated or tries to sit up, allow him/her to do so. The patient may be trying to cough up a foreign body, an indication of aspiration.

4. If the patient shows no evidence of respiratory obstruction and/or appears to have swallowed the foreign body, alert the Oral Surgery Emergency Team.

5. Instruct the patient to watch for the passage of the object and try to recover it. If it is not recovered, periodic films should be taken until there is evidence that the object has passed.

6. The clinician should obtain the Accident Reporting and Treatment Form and fill it out. This should be filed in the patient's chart.

Treatment

- Bronchoscopy and esophagoscopy
- immediate complications - acute airway obstruction and hypoxia, chronic complications – oesophageal erosion and pneumonia
- Bronchoscopy (flexible or rigid under general anaesthesia) is the treatment of choice for the removal of a foreign body
- For the removal of objects lodged in very small bronchi close to the lung parenchyma, fluoroscopic guidance can be used.

DENTOLEGAL CONSEQUENCES

Endodontic errors sometimes have dentolegal consequences. These can be minimised or avoided by providing patients with adequate information prior to the endodontic procedure and getting informed consent from the patient.

Documentation is essential to attain endodontic excellence. The dental record must contain sufficient information to identify the patient, support the diagnosis, justify the treatment and document the course and result of treatment.

The treatment complications in endodontics are relatively low among specialists compared to non-specialists. A retrospective study done by the Southwest Endodontic Society states that a reasonable endodontist or a practitioner with similar abilities should disclose the following facts to the patients:

- Endodontic therapy cannot be guaranteed.
- Although endodontic therapy is usually successful, a small percentage of teeth are lost despite competent endodontic care because of complications or treatment failure.
- Slight overextending or under-filling of root canals occurs in 2% to 4% of cases, which may contribute to treatment failure.
- Slight to moderate transient postoperative pain may occur. Severe postoperative pain rarely occurs.
- Irreparable damage to the existing crown or restoration secondary treatment is uncommon after the access opening is restored.

When a procedural accident occurs, the patient should be informed about the nature of the error, what can be done to correct it and what effect the error may have on the tooth's prognosis and on the entire treatment plan. If a procedural accident leads to a situation that is beyond the treating dentist's training and ability to handle, he or she should recognise the need to refer the patient to a specialist. It is important to note that the standard of care in endodontics is only one level; both general dentists and specialists are held to the same standard.

CONCLUSION

Procedural errors can be prevented, but only when we give every step the attention it deserves. Every error carries a lesson, and every lesson has the power to improve the next treatment. The literature is rich with experience, and the wise clinician learns not only from personal mistakes but also from the mistakes of others. When an error occurs, it should not be dismissed or hidden; it should be examined honestly, step by step, so that its cause is understood and its recurrence prevented.

Dentistry is more than a technical profession; it is a promise of trust. Patients place their confidence in us because they believe we will protect their health with skill, care, and integrity. That trust is earned not by speed, but by excellence. It is earned by patience, precision, and the courage to take an extra moment when needed to do the right thing.

Mistakes may be easy to make, but they are also easy to prevent when we practice with discipline and purpose. The true mark of a clinician is not whether complications ever happen, but how committed one is to avoiding them. Careful practice today prevents regret tomorrow. In the end, excellence is built not on haste, but on thoughtful action, constant learning, and unwavering respect for the patient.

REFERENCE

1. John Ide Ingle, Textbook of Endodontics, Fifth edition 2002, Leif K Bakland, Endodontic errors; 769-794.
2. James L Gutmann, Problem solving in endodontics – prevention, identification and management; 69-156.
3. Justman BC, Krell KV, A safe technique for removal of provisionally cemented crowns, J Endod 1993;19:97-8.
4. Alhadainy HA et al, Evaluation of the sealing ability of amalgam, cavity, and glass ionomer cement in the repair of furcation perforations, Oral Surg 1993; 75: 362.
5. ElDeeb ME, ElDeeb M, Tabibi A, Jensen JR, An evaluation of the use of amalgam, Cavit, and calcium hydroxide in the repair of furcation perforations. J Endod 1982; 8:459-66.
6. Alhadainy HA, Abdalla AI, Artificial floor technique used for the repair of furcation perforations: a microleakage study, J Endod 1998;24:33-5.
7. Himel VT, Brady J Jr, Weir J Jr, Evaluation of repair of mechanical perforations of the pulp chamber floor using biodegradable tricalcium phosp-hate or calcium hydroxide, J Endod 1985;11:161-5.
8. Lee SJ, Monsef M, Torabinejad M, Sealing ability of a mineral trioxide aggregate for repair of lateral root perforations, J Endod Nov;19:541-4.
9. Torabinejad M, Chivian N, Clinical applications of mineral trioxide aggregate, J Endod 1999 ;25:197-205.
10. Torabinejad M, Hong CU, McDonald F, Pitt Ford TR, Physical and chemical properties of a new root-end filling material, J Endod 1995;21:349-53.
11. Torabinejad M, Rastegar AF, Kettering JD, Pitt Ford TR, Bacterial leakage of mineral trioxide aggregate as a root-end filling material, J Endod 1995;21:109-12.
12. Fuss Z et al, Determination of location of root perforation using electronic apex locators, Oral surg 1996; 82:324.
13. ElDeeb ME, ElDeeb M, Tabibi A, Jensen JR, An evaluation of the use of amalgam, Cavit, and calcium hydroxide in the repair of furcation perforations. J Endod 1982;8:459-66 .
14. Eleazer PD, McDonald TW, Sinai IH, Fantasia JE, Michelich RJ, Yagiela JA, Proplast as an apical barrier in root canal therapy, J Endod 1984;10:487-90.
15. Goon WW, Lundergan WP, Redemption of a perforated furcation with a multidiscip-linary treatment approach, J Endod 1992;18:545-8.

16. Berutti E, Fedon G, Thickness of cementum/dentin in mesial roots of mandibular first molars, J Endod 1995;21:576-9.
17. Samuel I Kratchman, DCNA, Modern endodontic practice, Perforation repair and one step apexification procedures; 291-308.
18. Eleazer PD, McDonald TW, Sinai IH, Fantasia JE, Michelich RJ, Yagiela JA, Proplast as an apical barrier in root canal therapy, J Endod 1984;10:487-90.
19. Kim S et al, DCNA,1997, Hemostasis in endodontic microsurgery.
20. Haasch GC, Gerstein H, Austin BP, Effects of two hemostatic agents on osseous healing, J Endod 1989;15:310-4.
21. Cohen and Hargreaves, Pathways of the Pulp, 9th edition, 2006; 748-768.
22. Hartwell GR, England MC, Healing of furcation perforations in primate teeth after repair with decalcified freeze-dried bone: a longitudinal study, J Endod 1993;19:357-61.
23. Nakata TT, Bae KS, Baumgartner JC, Perforation repair comparing mineral trio-xide aggregate and amalgam using an anaerobic bacterial leakage model, J Endod 1998; 24:184-6.
24. Sluyk SR, Moon PC, Hartwell GR, Evaluation of setting properties and retention characteristics of mineral trioxide aggregate when used as a furcation perforation repair material, J Endod 1998;24:768-71.
25. O'Connor RP, Hutter JW, Roahen JO, Leakage of amalgam and Super-EBA root-end fillings using two preparation techniques and surgical microscopy, J Endod 1995; 21:74-8.
26. Arnold JW, Rueggeberg FA, Anderson RW, Weller RN, Borke JL, Pashley DH, The disintegration of super EBA cement in solutions with adjusted pH and osmolarity, J Endod 1997;23:663-8.
27. Harrison JW, Johnson SA, Excisional wound healing following the use of IRM as a root-end filling material, J Endod 1997;23:19-27.
28. Vignaroli PA, Anderson RW, Pashley DH, Longitudinal evaluation of the microleakage of dentin bonding agents used to seal resected root apices, J Endod. 1995;21:509-12.
29. Justman BC, Krell KV, A safe technique for removal of provisionally cemented crowns, J Endod 1993;19:97-8.
30. Andreasen JO, Munksgaard EC, Fredebo L, Rud J, Periodontal tissue regeneration including cementogenesis adjacent to dentin bonded retrograde composite fillings in humans, J Endod 1993;19:151-3.
31. Roane JB, Sabala CL, Duncanson MG Jr, The "balanced force" concept for instrumentation of curved canals, J Endod 1985;11:203-11.

32. Ralan Wong, DCNA, Modern endodontic practice, Conventional endodontic failure and retreatment; 265-290.
33. Hülsmann M, Removal of fractured instruments using a combined automated/ultrasonic technique, J Endod 1994; 20:144-7.
34. Jeff R. Ward, Peter Parashos, Harold H. Messer, Evaluation of an Ultrasonic Technique to Remove Fractured Rotary Nickel-Titanium Endodontic Instruments from Root Canals: An Experimental Study, J Endod 2003; 29: 756-763.
35. Gettleman BH, Spriggs KA, ElDeeb ME, Messer HH, Removal of canal obstructions with the endo extractor, J Endod 1998;24:446-8.
36. Sabala CL, Roane JB, Southard LZ, Instrumentation of curved canals using a modified tipped instrument: a comparison study, J Endod 1988;14:59-64.
37. N. Cohenca, I. Rotstein, Mental nerve paresthesia associated with a non-vital tooth, Endod dent traumatol 1996; 12: 298–300.
38. Pyner DA, Paresthesia of the inferior alveolar nerve caused by Hydron: a case report, J Endod. 1980;6:527-8.
39. Hayashi M, Kinomoto Y, Takeshige F, Ebisu S, Prognosis of intentional replantation of vertically fractured roots reconstructed with dentin-bonded resin, J Endod 2004; 30:145-8.
40. Sugaya T, Kawanami M, Noguchi H, Kato H, Masaka N, Periodontal healing after bonding treatment of vertical root fracture, Dent Traumatol 2001;17:174-9.
41. Trope M, Rosenberg ES, Multidisciplinary approach to the repair of vertically fractured teeth, J Endod 1992;18:460-3.
42. K Kawai, N Masaka, Vertical root fracture treated by bonding fragments and rotational replantation, Dent Traumatol; 18:42-5.
43. Tidmarsh BG, Restoration of endodontically treated posterior teeth, J Endod 1976;2:374-5.
44. Ehrich DG, Brian JD Jr, Walker WA, Sodium hypochlorite accident: inadvertent injection into the maxillary sinus, J Endod 1993; 19:180-2.
45. Bhat KS, Tissue emphysema caused by hydrogen peroxide, Oral Surg Oral Med Oral Pathol 1974;38:304-7.
46. Pashley EL, Birdsong NL, Bowman K, Pashley DH, Cytotoxic effects of NaOCl on vital tissue, J Endod 1985; 11:525-8.
47. Gatot A, Arbelle J, Leiberman A, Yanai-Inbar I, Effects of sodium hypochlorite on soft tissues after its inadvertent injection beyond the root apex, J Endod 1991;17:573-4.

48. Herrmann JW, Heicht RC, Complications in therapeutic use of sodium hypochlorite, J Endod 1979;5:160.
49. Hülsmann M, Hahn W, Complications during root canal irrigation – literature review and case reports, Int Endod J 2000; 33: 186–193.
50. Sabala CL, Powell SE, Sodium hypochlorite injection into periapical tissues, J Endod 1989; 15:490-2.
51. R. Witton, K. Henthorn, M. Ethunandan, S. Harmer & P. A. Brennan, Neurological complications following extrusion of sodium hypochlorite solution during root canal treatment, Int Endod J 2005; 38: 843-848.
52. Kaufman AY, Keila S, Hypersensitivity to sodium hypochlorite, J Endod 1989; 15:224-6.
53. Mejia JL, Donado JE, Posada A, Accidental swallowing of a dental clamp, J Endod 1996; 22:619-20.
54. Satheesh SL, Jain S, Bhuyan AC, Devi LS. Surgical management of a separated endodontic instrument using second-generation platelet concentrate and hydroxyapatite. Journal of clinical and diagnostic research: JCDR. 2017 Jun;11(6): ZD01

EPILOGUE

Every root canal treatment is an opportunity to restore health, relieve pain, and preserve a natural tooth. While procedural errors are an inevitable part of clinical practice, they should never define a clinician. Instead, they should be viewed as opportunities to learn, refine techniques, and grow professionally.

The true measure of an endodontist is not the absence of mistakes, but the ability to recognize them early, manage them effectively, and continuously strive for improvement. Excellence in endodontics is achieved through knowledge, precision, patience, and a commitment to lifelong learning.

I hope this book has provided practical guidance and strengthened your confidence in preventing and managing root canal errors. May it serve as a reliable companion throughout your clinical journey and inspire you to deliver the highest standard of patient care.

Remember, every challenge is an opportunity to become a better clinician, and every successful treatment reflects the dedication to learning and excellence.

Thank you for allowing this book to be a part of your professional journey.

Dr. Pavan Rajendra Tryambake

www.ingramcontent.com/pod-product-compliance
Lightning Source LLC
LaVergne TN
LVHW070936210926
848482LV00003B/258

* 9 7 9 8 9 0 5 8 4 1 6 1 3 *